CLINICAL PHYSIOLOGY MADE RIDICULOUSLY SIMPLE

Stephen Goldberg, M.D.
Associate Professor
Department of Cell Biology and Anatomy
University of Miami School of Medicine
Miami, Florida 33101

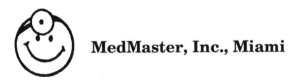

MedMaster, Inc., Miami

Made in the United States of America

Published by MedMaster, Inc.
P.O. Box 640028
Miami, FL 33164

Cover by Steve Goldberg and Jennifer Graeber

TO RUBE GOLDBERG, MASTER OF THE SEQUENTIAL REACTION

PREFACE

Physiology, the study of function of the components of living organisms, is perhaps the most important of the basic medical sciences, in view of the vast amount of physiological knowledge one has to use in everyday medical practice. I wrote this book to fulfill the need for a brief text that would provide a rapid, coherent view of the most important clinical principles and points in physiology. The book is intended for medical students but should also be of practical value to nurses and paramedical personnel who require a knowledge of physiology in their everyday medical practice.

Although there are many excellent reference texts in physiology, the student is commonly overwhelmed with detail and enters the wards in the third and fourth years with a fragmented knowledge of isolated facts. It is educationally more sound to first grasp overall concepts and key points and then to add supplementary details as time allows. The student commonly cannot do this when studying only from reference texts. One needs both the detailed reference and the brief book that presents the conceptual whole. Whatever time remains after first learning the overall principles can then be devoted to greater depth and breadth, and the learning will then be more rapid and permanent.

There is a close interrelationship between the many body systems, which make it difficult to isolate one system out of context of the others. This is particularly true of the circulatory system. Adequate tissue nutrition depends on the coordination of cardiac, pulmonary, and renal physiology, which influence blood pressure, blood volume, cardiac output, vascular caliber, and the chemical composition of the blood. A change in any of these may result in changes in the others, and a discussion of any one leads to the rest. The conceptual unification of these areas of physiology can be difficult to achieve when plodding through a long reference text. However, I attempt this unification in this book through brevity and emphasis on clinically relevant points.

Much of this book will be considered "incomplete" in view of the vast body of physiological knowledge. A number of points that may be functionally important but clinically unimportant are underemphasized, whereas clinically important points are emphasized even if they may not be the most important functionally, or stressed in other physiology books. As physiology overlaps into biochemistry, cell biology, anatomy, and other subjects, I have had to judge where to make the cutoffs, as it would become too unwieldy to intrude too deeply into the other fields. I hope that what has emerged will provide a valuable link to the other fields and make learning easier and more enjoyable.

National Boards now emphasize clinically relevant material, and the material presented in this book should provide the most important information relevant to Board study.

I thank Drs. David Adams, Raul De Gasperi, Joan Mayer, Lincoln Potter, Richard Preston, and Beverly Vollenhoven, for their advice on many clinical and physiologic points in this book, and Phyllis Goldenberg for editing the manuscript. I was fortunate to find Steve Goldberg (no relation) who, as a medical student at the University of Miami, drew many of the humorous but educationally pertinent illustrations. These were complimented with artwork by Jennifer Graeber, a superb medical illustrator. I take full credit for the remaining illustrations of lower quality.

Stephen Goldberg

CONTENTS

PART I: CARDIO-PULMONARY-RENAL-ELECTROLYTE-ACID-BASE-BALANCE

CHAPTER 1. CELL FUNCTION

Certain functions occur in all cells, whereas others occur only in specialized cells in particular organs.

Fig. 1-1. The intracellular localization of biochemical reactions.

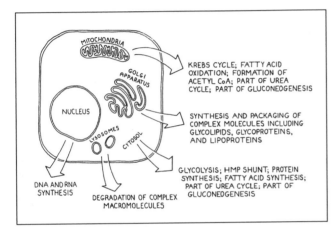

KREBS CYCLE; FATTY ACID OXIDATION; FORMATION OF ACETYL CoA; PART OF UREA CYCLE; PART OF GLUCONEOGENESIS

SYNTHESIS AND PACKAGING OF COMPLEX MOLECULES INCLUDING GLYCOLIPIDS, GLYCOPROTEINS, AND LIPOPROTEINS

GLYCOLYSIS; HMP SHUNT; PROTEIN SYNTHESIS; FATTY ACID SYNTHESIS; PART OF UREA CYCLE; PART OF GLUCONEOGENESIS

DNA AND RNA SYNTHESIS

DEGRADATION OF COMPLEX MACROMOLECULES

MITOCHONDRIA, GOLGI APPARATUS, NUCLEUS, LYSOSOMES, CYTOSOL

Figure 1-1

Fig. 1-2. The organ localization of some key biochemical reactions.

The cell membrane accounts for some of the major differences between cells. Many cells contain specialized cell surface receptors that enable selective recognition of those cells by hormones and other cells. For instance, thyroid stimulating hormone (TSH) affects thyroid cells because thyroid cells contain receptors for TSH.

A very important part of cell function that relates to cell physiology is the mechanism that controls the entry into cells of simple molecules, like sodium and potassium ions. If such molecules entered cells only by simple diffusion, then the intra-and extracellular milieu would contain the same concentrations of these molecules, whereas radically different intra- and extracellular concentrations are necessary for life.

Fig. 1-3. The major mechanisms of transport of chemicals across cell membranes:

1) **Simple diffusion** along the molecule's electrochemical concentration gradient. That is, molecules tend to move from a zone in which their concentration is higher to a zone in which their concentration is lower. Similar reasoning applies when there is a charge imbalance between two zones, in which case an ion will tend to move so as to equalize the charges. Increased pressure on the molecules that are to diffuse across a membrane will also increase the tendency to diffuse, by increasing the concentration and/or the kinetic energy of the diffusing molecule.

Simple diffusion, however, depends in large part on the permeability of the membrane across which the molecules diffuse. Regardless of the electrochemical gradient, diffusion will not occur if the membrane is nonpermeable to the molecule in question. Lipid-soluble (nonpolar) substances more readily diffuse across cell plasma membranes, whereas polar substances diffuse more readily through water-filled channels (e.g. Na+ and K+ channels) within the plasma membrane.

2) **Simple facilitated diffusion**. The molecule moves along its electrochemical concentration gradient, but it is attached to some other "carrier" protein molecule that facilitates its passage. For instance, a polar molecule may have difficulty passing through a lipid cell membrane, but it will do so more readily if attached to another molecule that passes easily. Whereas simple diffusion increases in proportion to the concentration of the diffusing molecule, simple facilitated diffusion reaches a maximum that depends on the concentration of the carrier molecule. Simple facilitated diffusion does not move against an electrochemical gradient, and no special energy input is necessary to drive it. (The process of simple facilitated diffusion does, however, release energy, which may dissipate as heat or be used for other purposes.)

3) **Primary active transport**. The molecule moves **against** its electrochemical concentration gradient, and the energy supplied for this comes from ATP, which is the "energy currency" of the body. For instance, the pumping of sodium against its gradient, out of a renal tubular cell and into the peritubular capillaries, requires a Na/K ATPase, an enzyme that converts ATP to ADP to release energy.

4) **Secondary active transport**. As in primary active transport, the molecule moves against its electro-

---

HOUSEKEEPING (GENERALIZED) ORGAN FUNCTIONS

Fatty acid oxidation (*)(**)
Glycolysis
Glycogen synthesis and breakdown
Krebs cycle and oxidative phosphorylation (**)
Protein synthesis (**)

(*) except in brain
(**) except in mature red blood cells

SPECIALIZED ORGAN FUNCTIONS	**MAJOR SITES**
Fatty acid synthesis	liver, fat cells
Gluconeogenesis	liver, kidney
Heme synthesis	bone marrow
HMP shunt	liver, fat cells, adrenal cortex mammary gland, red blood cells
Amino acid synthesis and breakdown	liver
Urea synthesis	liver
Cholesterol and bile acid synthesis	liver
Steroid hormone synthesis	adrenal cortex, gonads

Figure 1-2

---

chemical concentration gradient. However, the energy supplied for this does not come directly from ATP; instead, energy comes from the movement of another molecule along its electrochemical gradient. For instance, glucose, amino acids, phosphate, and other molecules undergo secondary active transport from the renal tubular lumen into renal tubule cells against their concentration gradients (with the assistance of carrier molecules), using energy derived from simple diffusion of sodium into the cell along its electrochemical gradient. The situation is somewhat analogous to energy from falling water (sodium diffusion) turning a water wheel (glucose transport). In the case of glucose, this normally results in virtual removal of all glucose in the proximal renal tubule. This does not mean that all the glucose is always going to be reabsorbed in the kidney. If there is too great a concentration of glucose, the system is over-whelmed (i.e. it has reached its transport maximum, or "Tm") and some may not be reabsorbed. Glucose, normally absent from the urine, commonly appears in the urine when its blood concentration reaches about 180 mg/dL.

Cotransport is secondary active transport in which the transported molecule (moving uphill against its gradient) and the molecule supplying the energy (moving downhill along its gradient) are moving in the same direction across the membrane. In **countertransport**, they move in opposite directions (Fig. 1-3).

5) **Endocytosis**. Endocytosis involves an invagination of the plasma membrane to encompass and take in the transported material. It is a way of transporting macromolecules, such as proteins. Endocytosis is actually a form of active transport as it uses ATP as an energy source.

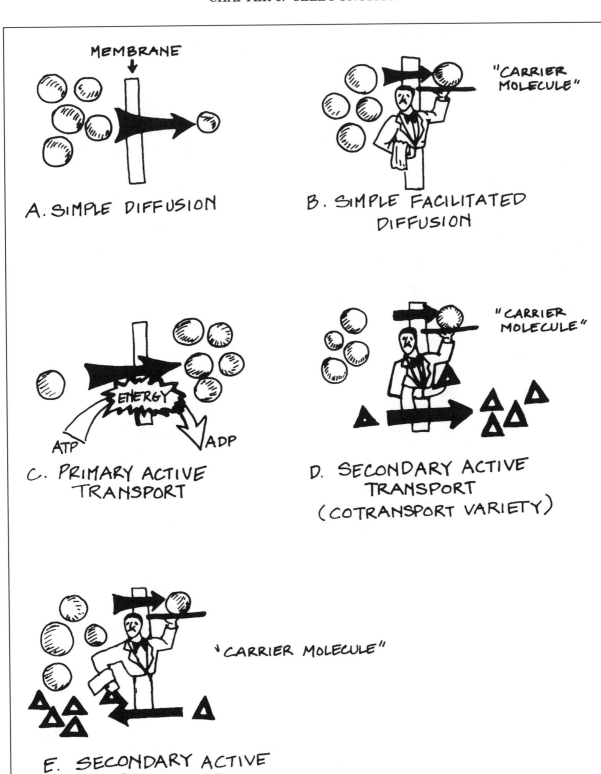

Figure 1-3

CHAPTER 2. BLOOD PRESSURE

Homeostasis

Homeostasis is the tendency for the body to maintain itself in a stable state. Many control mechanisms accomplish this. For instance, at the biochemical level, end products of a chemical reaction chain may feed back to the beginning of the chain to suppress an overproduction of the end product. Buffers prevent the body pH from changing too radically. Negative feedback loops in the neuronal circuitry prevent the impulses along a neural pathway from having too much of an effect. Rather than rote memorization of the reactions of the body to all kinds of stress (which will increase your own stress), you can save a lot of studying time by appreciating, logically, that in just about all areas of body function there are homeostatic mechanisms that will do what one would expect: namely, act efficiently to prevent reactions from going too far and to restore stability to body function. Such mechanisms are especially prominent in the interactions of the cardiovascular, renal, and pulmonary systems.

What Is Blood Pressure?

In the usual context, blood pressure refers to brachial artery pressure, which in the average adult is about 120/80. The "120" (in mm Hg) refers to **systolic pressure**, the brachial arterial pressure during cardiac ventricular contraction. The "80" is **diastolic pressure**, the brachial arterial pressure during cardiac ventricular relaxation. The average between the two, thus, is about 100. Such an average of 100 may be abnormal if the pulse difference (termed the **arterial pulse pressure**) is wide. For instance:

1) A pressure of 160/40 for which the average is also 100, may occur in **arteriosclerosis,** wherein hardening of the arteries permits little flexibility of the vessels. The pressure then may dramatically rise in systole, due to vascular rigidity, and dramatically fall back in diastole.

2) In **aortic regurgitation,** where blood flows backward through an incompetent aortic valve, the diastolic pressure may be low, due to the runoff of blood back to the heart, whereas the systolic pressure may be elevated due to the added volume of (the returned) blood that the heart has to pump with each beat.

3) **Patent ductus arteriosus** (Fig. 2-1). Before birth, blood largely bypasses the lungs and flows from the pulmonary artery directly into the aorta via the ductus arteriosus, because the collapsed lungs resist pulmonary blood flow; the fetus does not oxygenate its blood via the lungs. Normally the ductus closes after birth. If this does not occur, blood flows from the aorta

redundantly into the pulmonary circulation. This backflow causes an attempt to increase the cardiac output, with limited tolerance to exercise. In each diastole of patent ductus, there is relatively little resistance to blood flow, as blood, in addition to its normal flow down the aorta, also runs back into the pulmonary circulation, thereby reducing diastolic pressure. The extra volume that the heart then has to pump out during systole results in a higher systolic pressure.

Fig. 2-1. Patent ductus arteriosus.

Fig. 2-2. Mean blood pressure* varies in different parts of the circulation, being about 100 in the major arteries where it is usually tested, and close to 0 where the venae cava enter the heart. This progressive drop

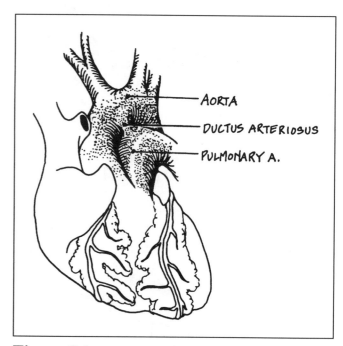

Figure 2-1

in mean blood pressure is the result of resistance to blood flow, **particularly at the arteriolar level**, where the vessels narrow to become capillaries. By the time blood has reached the capillaries, mean blood pressure is down to about 30mm Hg. The difference in

---

*The term "mean arterial blood pressure" means something slightly different from the average between the sys-

4

MEAN BLOOD PRESSURE (mm Hg)	
Aorta and Large Arteries	100
Arterioles	35–80
Capillaries	10–35
Venules	5–10
Vena Cava and Right Atrium	0–2
Pulmonary Artery	16
Pulmonary Capillaries and Left Atrium	7

Figure 2-2

pressure between the arteries (100) and the end of the vena caval system (about 0) is very important to blood flow as it is the pressure **difference** that mediates blood flow. If mean pressure were 100 throughout the vascular system, there would be no flow at all. You could pump up a cadaver's circulatory system to the bursting level and then stop to observe. No blood flow would result from the uniformly increased pressure, because blood flows only from an area of higher pressure to an an area of lower pressure.

In a standing person, mean blood pressure in the arteries and veins is significantly higher in the feet than in the upper extremities because of the added weight of the blood (e.g. 100 mm Hg in the brachial artery and 180 mm Hg in the arteries of the feet). Muscular activity of the lower extremities helps prevent venous pressure from rising too high in the feet. The veins contain one-way valves that keep blood flowing toward the heart, and muscular activity propels the blood past the valves, reducing the pooling of blood in the feet. Incompetent valves may result in blood pooling, with varicose veins and edema of the feet.

Measurement Of Blood Pressure

Usually blood pressure is measured by inflating a blood pressure cuff over the arm and listening with the stethescope over the brachial artery at the brachial fossa. Normally, with no cuff, there are no audible sounds. When the cuff is inflated beyond the systolic pressure, there certainly is no sound heard, because no blood can get through the brachial artery. When the cuff is slowly deflated to just below the systolic

tolic and diastolic pressure. It is the average of many pressure samplings during a given cardiac cycle. Since more samples lie closer to the diastolic pressure than to the systolic pressure during a given cycle, the mean arterial blood pressure is slightly closer to the diastolic than to the systolic pressure.

pressure, blood passes with each systole, but the arteries collapse again during diastole. This fluctuation of blood flow causes the **Korotkoff sounds** that are heard during blood pressure recording. As you deflate the cuff, the pressure when the Kortokoff sounds first appear is the **systolic pressure.** The point of disappearance of the sounds is the **diastolic pressure,** the point at which the diastolic pressure equals the cuff pressure, enabling blood to pass during both systole and diastole.

What's So Important About Blood Pressure?

Without blood pressure, you die quickly, as pressure is necessary to drive blood flow (**perfusion**) through the tissues. With blood pressure that is too high, you may die acutely: a blood vessel may burst suddenly, causing a stroke (loss of circulation to a portion of the brain); or there may be longer-range problems, such as arteriosclerosis. The body has developed multiple mechanisms to ensure the proper control of blood pressure.

What Controls the Blood Pressure?

Fig. 2-3. The key factors that regulate systemic blood pressure are **peripheral resistance**—particularly as mediated through blood vessel constriction (vasoconstriction)—and **cardiac output** (heart stroke volume x heart rate, normally about 5–6 liters/min). An increase in either of these factors will increase blood pressure.

Increased **peripheral resistance** raises pressure by impeding blood flow, resulting in backup of blood in the arteries, where blood pressure is measured. Resistance increases mainly through vasoconstriction, particularly at the arteriolar level, but may also increase somewhat through elevated friction in cases of increased blood viscosity.

Cardiac output is extremely important in determining blood pressure, for if the heart were to suddenly stop, with no change in overall blood volume or peripheral resistance, the blood pressure would drop to about 5–10 mm Hg (the **mean circulatory filling pressure,** the pressure one would find if the heart were to stop). The reason is that heart contraction forces a bolus (localized collection) of blood into the arterial system, stretching the arterial walls and raising the arterial pressure significantly during systole. This local pressure is then transmitted down the vascular tree, because blood moves from an area of high pressure to an area of lower pressure.

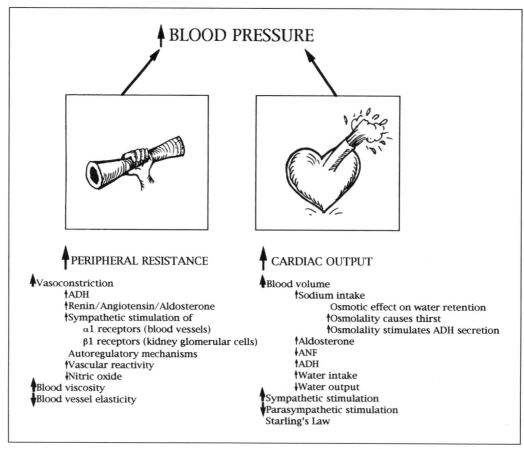

Figure 2-3

In normal individuals, the increase in cardiac output associated with exercise is mainly associated with a rise in systolic, rather than diastolic, pressure. In athletes, an increased cardiac output may be associated with a relatively low pressure, suggesting that their vascular resistance may be relatively low during exercise.

Increasing the **blood volume** increases pressure by increasing cardiac output. Blood volume is partly a function of the balance of fluid intake and output. Output occurs mainly through the kidneys, and to a much lesser extent, through the skin, lungs, and digestive tract. Blood volume also depends significantly on osmotic and other forces that tend to keep fluid within the blood vessels, as opposed to the extravascular spaces.

Fig. 2-4. Fluid intake and loss through skin, lungs, and digestive tract.

Blood volume changes directly with the body levels of sodium, as sodium is the most abundant of the plasma electrolytes; this gives sodium a powerful osmotic effect

INTAKE	mL/Day
Food	2200
Body Metabolism	300
TOTAL	2500
OUTPUT	
Kidney	1500
Skin/Lungs	925
GI Tract	75
TOTAL	2500

Figure 2-4

in retaining water. Water tends to follow where sodium goes. Increased plasma sodium results in increased water retention. Normal adult blood volume is about 5–6 liters.

Not shown in Fig. 2-3 is the important point that blood pressure is also controlled by negative feedback of blood pressure itself. That is, decreased (or increased) blood pressure stimulates a homeostatic increase (or decrease) in blood pressure. Similar negative feedback mechanisms exist for peripheral resistance, cardiac output, and blood volume. Each entity feeds back to regulate itself in addition to influencing all the others.

The body has many intertwining mechanisms to detect and respond to changes in blood pressure, blood volume, peripheral resistance, and cardiac output, which will herewith be discussed as a whole. Receptors in the nervous system, kidney, heart, and peripheral vasculature play important roles in circulatory control:

1) **Receptors in the nervous system**

Both the brain stem and hypothalamus contain blood pressure regulating centers.

The brain stem contains a vasomotor center (influenced by numerous other areas of the nervous system), which increases blood pressure by firing sympathetic nerve messages (see Chapter 9, Neurophysiology, for further information on the sympathetic nervous system). Sympathetic nerves release norepinephrine, which stimulates **alpha-1** receptors on the peripheral blood vessels (causing vasoconstriction) as well as **beta-1** receptors on heart muscle (increasing cardiac output by increasing both stroke volume and heart rate). As veins contain most of the body's blood (largely for blood storage), the vasoconstrictive effect on the venous system can be particularly important in restoring blood pressure; venous constriction helps restore effective arterial blood volume in the rest of the body following fluid loss (as in hemorrhage). The veins hold about two thirds of the body's blood (the arteries and arterioles about 15%, and the capillaries only about 5%).

Sympathetic nerves also stimulate the **adrenal medulla** to secrete both **norepinephrine and epinephrine**, which reach the entire body through the circulation. No**R**epinephrine, present also in sympathetic nerve endings, has ge**Ne**ral vasoconstrictive effects, by interacting with blood vessel **alpha-1** receptors. Epinephrine vasoconstricts too, but not in all places. Like norepinephrine, epinephrine causes vasoconstriction when it acts on blood vessel alpha-1 receptors, but vasodilation when it acts on blood vessel **beta-2** receptors, most notably those in skeletal muscle and heart. (The "**B**" in Beta stand for "**B**igger diameter vessel"—not really.)

Norepinephrine does not act on beta-2 receptors. Thus it is logical to understand that sympathetic nerve endings, which rely on norepinephrine to transmit messages, do not innervate beta-2 receptors. Freely circulating epinephrine, however, does stimulate beta-2 receptors and thereby dilates skeletal and heart coronary blood vessels. This helps to ensure perfusion of the latter organs in states of sympathetic activity, as in the flight-or-fight response, where increased cardiac and skeletal circulation is critical.

Fig. 2-5. Location and effects of stimulation of adrenergic receptors.

Sympathetic nerves stimulate **beta-1** receptors on cardiac muscle, including the modified muscle cells of the SA and AV nodes, which are part of the pacemaker and conduction system of the heart. This stimulation increases heart rate, conduction velocity through the AV node, and cardiac muscle contractility, with a net increase in cardiac output.

In addition, sympathetic nerves stimulate beta-1 receptors on granular cells in the kidney to cause renin secretion. Renin initiates a chain reaction that results in the production of angiotensin II and aldosterone. Both angiotensin II and aldosterone have powerful vasoconstrictive effects and, in addition, stimulate the renal tubules to reabsorb sodium (and, passively, water), thereby increasing pressure and blood volume.

The direct effect of the sympathetic nervous system on vasoconstriction throughout the body provides a more immediate control of blood pressure than does the longer range measure of altering blood volume through urine output.

The brain stem vasomotor center also contains a depressor region which connects with the parasympathetic system via the vagus nerve, thereby decreasing heart rate (and to some degree stroke volume) and, therefore, blood pressure when stimulated. Parasympathetic nerves do not significantly innervate peripheral blood vessels.

The hypothalamus releases **antidiuretic hormone (ADH)**. ADH acts on the kidney to increase water reabsorption from the renal tubules, thereby increasing blood volume and, hence, blood pressure. ADH also constricts blood vessels, thereby increasing peripheral resistance. Hence its other name—**vasopressin**.

The brain stem and hypothalamic centers are notified of the need for a change in blood pressure in several ways:

a) Venous, cardiac, and arterial **baroreceptors** (carotid and aortic sinuses) respond to a drop in blood pressure by reducing their normal rate of firing to the blood pressure centers in the brain stem and hypothalamus. Normally, baroreceptor firing INHIBITS the brain stem sympathetic center from issuing its sympathetic output (but stimulates the parasympathetic system), and INHIBITS the hypo-

LOCATION AND EFFECTS OF STIMULATION OF ADRENERGIC RECEPTORS	

ALPHA-1 RECEPTORS
 	
Arterioles and Veins:
  constriction (epinephrine and norepinephrine)
 	
Glands:
↓ secretions
 	
Eye:
  constriction of radial muscle
 	
Intestine:
↓ motility
	ALPHA-2 RECEPTORS
	
	CNS Postsynaptic Terminals:
	↓ sympathetic outflow from brain
	
	CNS Presynaptic Terminals:
	  norepinephrine release
	
	Beta Islet Cells of Pancreas:
	↓ secretion

BETA-1 RECEPTORS
 	
Heart:
↑ heart rate (SA node)
↑ contractility
↑ conduction velocity
↑ automaticity
 	
Kidney:
↑ renin secretion
	BETA-2 RECEPTORS
	
	Trachea and Bronchioles:
	  dilation
	
	Pregnant/nonpregnant Uterus:
	  relaxation
	
	Arterioles (no beta-2 receptors in skin or brain):
	  dilation (epinephrine)

Figure 2-5

thalamus from secreting ADH. Decreased blood pressure, then reduces baroreceptor firing. Decrease baroreceptor firing increases sympathetic outflow (and decreases parasympathetic outflow), with a consequent rise in blood pressure. Decreased blood pressure also acts, via decreased baroreceptor firing, to increase ADH secretion by the hypothalamus, which in turn also contributes to a rise in blood pressure by increasing vasoconstriction and fluid retention.

Fig. 2-6. Effect of blood pressure and pH on sympathetic output of the brain stem.

Fig. 2-7. Effect of blood pressure and osmolality on hypothalamic ADH secretion.

Prolonged bed rest (as well as prolonged weightlessness in space) promotes fluid loss, because the pressure of blood is shifted from the lower extremities (while standing) to the upper body, where the baroreceptors are. This stimulates the baroreceptors to institute a pressure-lowering sequence that includes the excretion of water.

Carotid sinus massage is sometimes used to control tachycardia (excessively rapid heart rate). The pressure on the carotid sinus stimulates it to send sympathetic-inhibiting (parasympathetic-stimulating) impulses to the brain stem.

b) **Increased serum osmolality** (mainly due to an increase in sodium) acts on the hypothalamus to increase ADH secretion. (**Osmolality** is a property of a solution that increases with an increase in the number of dissolved dissociated particles in the solution.) It is as if the body, through many years of evolution and adverse environmental circumstances, came to realize that increased serum osmolality commonly means dehydration and the need to restore blood volume and pressure. So the hypothalamus then secretes more ADH (Fig. 2-7). The hypothalamus also responds to serum hyperosmolality by inducing the perception of thirst and the behavioral activities needed to increase fluid input (i.e. taking a drink of water).

c) Increased blood **CO_2 and H^+** levels (as might occur with low blood pressure and resultant inadequate tissue perfusion) affect the brain stem, stimulating the vasomotor center in the brain stem to

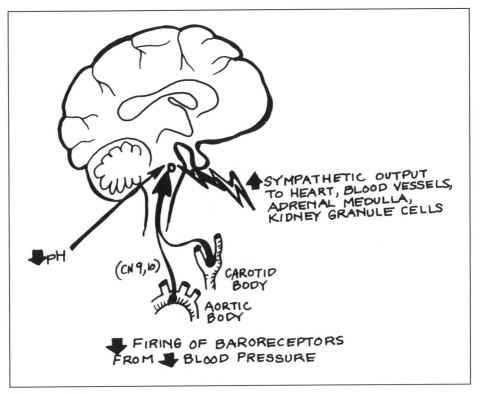

Figure 2-6

increase sympathetic output, thereby raising systemic blood pressure.

Diabetics frequently experience an excess production of urine (**polyuria**). One might expect that diabetics should experience the opposite—water retention—because of the hyperosmotic plasma, which is high in glucose and should stimulate ADH secretion. However, the osmotic effect of the excess glucose in the renal tubules prevents water from being reabsorbed into the peritubular capillaries and promotes water excretion.

A paradox: ADH retains water and enables the body to replace missing fluid. The stimulus for ADH secretion, though, is not low volume, but low blood pressure (as detected through the baroreceptors) and increased plasma hyperosmolality. What happens, then, if both plasma volume and osmolality are low (e.g. blood loss, with partial replacement with water)? One would like to increase the volume, but will not the low osmolality prevent this? The baroreceptors would indirectly detect the decreased volume (by virtue of the consequent decreased blood pressure) and serve to stimulate ADH secretion, but the low osmolality should **inhibit** ADH release. The actual final result will depend on which is worse, the volume or the osmolality abnormality. If the low extracellular fluid volume (manifest as decreased

blood pressure) is pronounced, then this influence will predominate toward restoring volume (and blood pressure) despite the hypoosmolality.

Alcohol inhibits ADH release, which may account for the increased diuresis following alcohol ingestion.

2) **Receptors in the kidney**

Changes in blood pressure and plasma osmolality affect blood pressure not only by influencing receptors in the nervous system, but also by influencing the kidney at the glomerular level and the level of the juxtaglomerular apparatus:

    a) **The glomerular level**. When blood passes through the kidney, a certain amount of water filters from the renal glomerular capillaries through the renal glomerular apparatus into the renal tubules.

Fig. 2-8. Overall view of the nephron.

Fig. 2-9. Schematic view of the renal corpuscle (= glomerulus + Bowman's capsule). A **glomerulus** is kind of a curled arterial portal system that stretches between the afferent (entering) and efferent (leaving) renal arterioles.

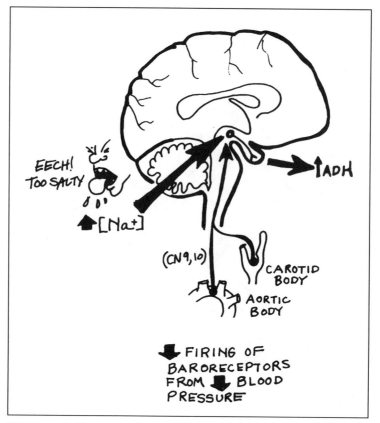

Figure 2-7

The ability of water to pass through the glomerular membrane depends largely on the blood's **hydraulic pressure**, its **osmotic pressure**, and the **surface area** and **permeability** of the glomerular membrane.

The hydraulic pressure of blood is the blood pressure. The higher the blood pressure, the more easily water will flow through the glomerular membrane to be excreted, because water flows from an area of high pressure to an area of lower pressure. More water filtration means reduced blood volume, an important way in which high blood pressure is reduced.

The osmotic pressure of a solution of relatively high osmolality refers to the tendency of water to be drawn into the solution. More technically, osmotic pressure is the hydraulic pressure necessary to keep water from entering the hyperosmotic solution through a membrane permeable only to water. Osmotic pressure of the plasma varies directly with its osmolality. The lower the plasma osmolality, the more dilute it is, and the greater is the filtration of water through the glomerular membrane into Bowman's space.

On the arteriolar end of a typical **nonrenal** capillary, water filters through the capillary wall just beyond the arteriole, because the hydraulic pressure drives it through. However, in the course of doing so, the intracapillary hydraulic pressure decreases while the intracapillary osmotic pressure increases and draws back fluid on the venous side of the capillary. Thus, there is little net loss of fluid into the interstitial tissues for the typical body capillary.

Plasma osmolality normally is higher than the osmolality of the glomerular filtrate, because proteins normally do not filter freely at the glomerular level, as do sodium and water. The relatively higher plasma osmolality tends to draw water back into the plasma rather than into the glomerulus, because molecules in general, including water, tend to diffuse between two regions so as to equalize their individual concentrations in both places. The net balance of hydraulic and osmotic pressures in the plasma and glomerular filtrate is key in determining the amount of water that is filtered. Thus, with decreased blood hydraulic pressure and increased plasma osmolality, less water will filter through the renal glomerulus, and fluid will be retained.

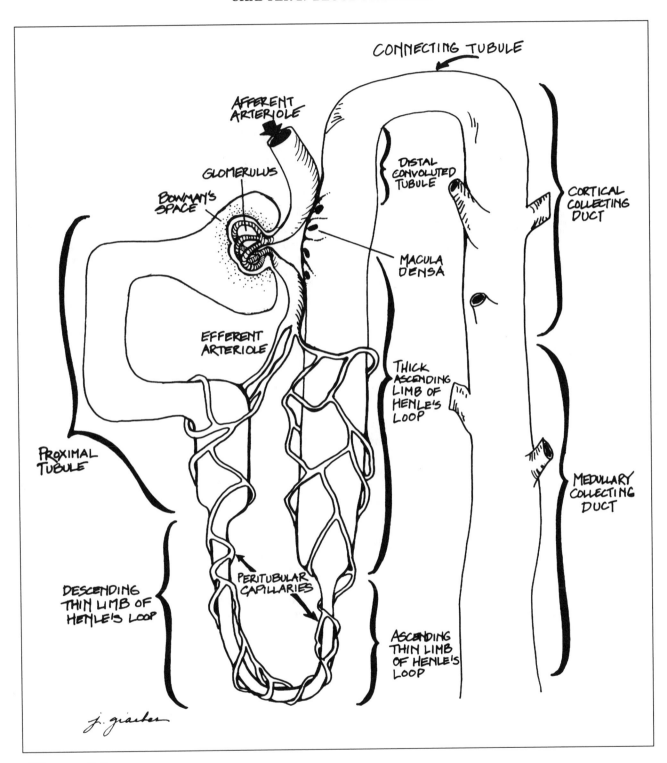

Figure 2-8

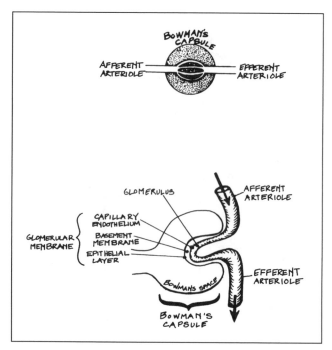

Figure 2-9

In addition to hydraulic and osmotic pressure of the blood, the ability of water to filter through the glomerular membrane depends on the surface area and permeability of the membrane. These may change in various diseases. The surface area of the vascular tuft in the glomerulus can decrease normally through the contraction of **mesangial cells**, which lie in the capillary loops of the glomerular capsule. ADH, as well as angiotensin II, promote the contraction of mesangial cells, thus providing a further mechanism of sodium and water retention via the reduction of fluid filtration into the nephron.

   b) **The juxtaglomerular apparatus** and the **renin-angiotensin-aldosterone pathway.** The juxtaglomerular apparatus includes the **granular cells** of the afferent arterioles, the **macula densa cells**, and extraglomerular **mesangial cells**.

Fig. 2-10. Sympathetic nerves stimulate the secretion of **renin** from the granular cells of the juxtaglomerular apparatus. Renin converts **angiotensinogen** (from the liver) to **angiotensin I. Angiotensin converting enzyme (ACE)** in the pulmonary capillaries converts angiotensin I to **angiotensin II**, which stimulates the secretion of **aldosterone** in the adrenal cortex. Aldosterone promotes the renal tubule reabsorption of sodium, with accompanying water, thereby increasing blood volume and pressure.

Low blood pressure also directly stimulates the granular cells to produce renin (via beta-1 adrenergic stimulation). In addition, there is a third mechanism that stimulates the granular cells in the afferent arteriolar wall. The **macula densa** is a region of the renal tubule that lies in apposition to the granular cells of the afferent arteriole. When the renal tubular fluid is low in sodium, the macula densa senses this and sends a message to the **granular cells** to release renin, which in turn leads to an increased absorption of sodium (via angiotensin II and aldosterone), and hence, to fluid retention and an increase in blood pressure. The way this works is as follows:

Most sodium (about 65%) is normally absorbed in the proximal renal tubule, leaving only a relatively small amount to be absorbed by the time the tubular fluid reaches the macula densa. **If blood volume is low**, fluid filtration through the glomerulus will slow, and there will be more time for sodium to be absorbed in the proximal tubule. Less sodium will reach the macula densa, which will detect this and act to restore fluid volume by stimulating renin secretion and increasing sodium reabsorption. Another reason why the tubular fluid at the macula densa might be low in sodium is that the body in itself might be **low in sodium**. The macula densa, in sensing this, stimulates renin secretion, which will increase sodium reabsorption.

Fig. 2-11. Sites of molecular uptake and secretion by the kidney tubules (further explained in Chapter 3).

When the plasma sodium concentration is abnormally high, how should the body look at this—as there being too much sodium or too little water in the body? That is, should the body act to increase sodium excretion or promote water retention? Interestingly, the hypothalamus, when faced with a hyperosmolar plasma, acts to increase water retention, via ADH, whereas the kidney acts to excrete more sodium via a decrease in the renin-angiotensin-aldosterone axis. The osmotic balance of the plasma depends on separate but interacting mechanisms that control sodium or water balance.

   c) **Prostaglandins.** Although renin hogs most of the limelight, it is important to note that the kidney also produces vasodilatory and vasoconstrictor lipids—prostaglandins—that may have important regulatory effects on blood pressure. The prostaglandins may be produced in interstitial cells that lie between the renal tubules and peritubular capillaries.

3) **Receptors in the heart**

   a) **Atrial natriuretic factor (ANF).** The atrial walls respond to stretch (i.e. to increased fluid volume) by the release of ANF, which acts on the renal

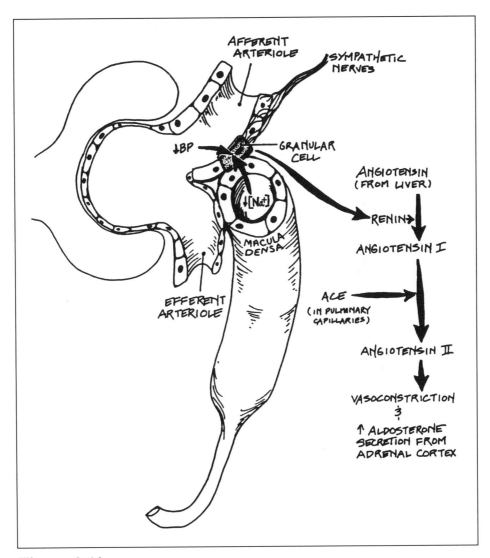

Figure 2-10

tubular system to promote sodium excretion and, passively, water excretion, thereby reducing plasma fluid volume. ANF increases glomerular filtration rate by eliciting vasodilation of the afferent arteriole and relaxing the glomerular mesangial cells. It also inhibits the following: plasma renin activity, sodium reabsorption particularly in the medullary collecting duct, and the synthesis and release of aldosterone. All of these activities of ANF result in reduced blood volume and blood pressure.

b) **Starling's law.** Cardiac output depends on both stroke volume and heart rate. Stroke volume depends not only on the degree of sympathetic cardiac stimulation, but on the blood volume. According to Starling's law, the greater the stretch on the car-

diac wall (i.e., the greater the volume entering a cardiac chamber), the greater will be the cardiac contraction in response to stretch. This occurs even without sympathetic nerve connections. Starling's law enables the heart to increase its output in accord with its input.

4) **Local receptors in the peripheral vasculature**

Apart from neuronal innervation and freely circulating chemical factors, local chemicals have a significant effect on the state of vasoconstriction. Arteriolar dilation occurs, letting more blood through to the tissues, if the metabolic needs of the tissues increase, as in exercise or inflammation. The affected tissues produce factors

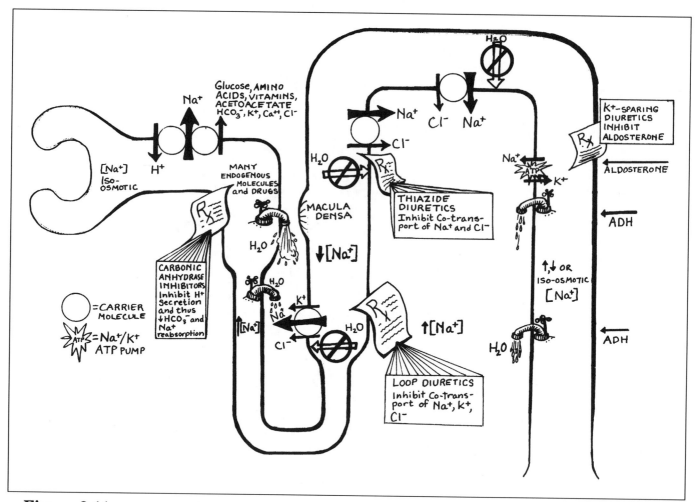

Figure 2-11

(CO₂, lactic acid, hydrogen, potassium and magnesium ions, adenosine, bradykinin, histamine) that dilate the arterioles locally. Simple increased plasma osmolality causes local arteriolar vasodilation. Also, the lack of O₂ may result in vasodilation, because O₂ itself helps maintain muscular contraction of the arteriolar wall. Conversely, excess blood flow through the tissues will tend to cause vasoconstriction through this "autoregulative effect." Whereas sympathetic innervation acts on the arterioles, the autoregulative effect actually acts on more peripheral extensions of the arterioles, termed metarterioles, which lie between the arterioles and capillaries.

Interestingly, in the lung, autoregulation has an opposite effect. Low alveolar oxygen concentration results in local vasoconstriction. This helps to ensure that blood is diverted from poorly aerated areas of the lung to areas better able to supply oxygen. In atelectasis (collapse of part of the lung), the collapse in itself serves to mechanically constrict blood vessels, so that blood flow is diverted to better aerated areas.

Calcium, which is important in stimulating muscle contraction, causes vasoconstriction. Prostaglandins are spread diffusely throughout the tissues of the body. Some of them cause vasodilation and others vasoconstriction. Serotonin, concentrated in platelets and in chromaffin cells in the abdomen, may have vasoconstrictive or vasodilatory effects.

Autoregulation of peripheral blood vessels provides an immediate response to tissue anoxia (oxygen deprivation). A longer-range response consists of an increase in blood vessel number and size, through the local production of an angiogenesis factor.

Something akin to Starling's law of the heart may also apply to the peripheral vasculature. When blood vessel walls are stretched, there is local vasoconstriction, which protects the capillary bed from acutely and excessively high blood pressure.

Last but not least, a growing literature indicates a very important role for **nitric oxide** in the regulation of blood pressure. Nitric oxide normally is found in vascular endothelium. It causes vasodilation, which may be an important reason why nitroglycerin is effective in increasing coronary dilation in response to angina. Nitric oxide becomes deficient with arteriosclerosis, providing another mechanism for pathological vasoconstriction, other than the arteriosclerosis itself.

When Things Go Wrong

As we have seen, the body has multiple control mechanisms to maintain blood pressure. These work fine to maintain homeostasis, unless there are marked stresses on the system or if individual components of the system are not working. For instance:

1) **Marked fluid loss**, through hemorrhage, diarrhea, vomiting, or sweating may severely strain the ability of the body to compensate and return blood volume to normal.

2) **Renal disease**. A normally functioning kidney usually suffices to excrete excess water and sodium, but water and sodium intake must be carefully regulated if the kidneys are malfunctioning (e.g. through intrinsic renal disease or renal artery stenosis). Otherwise, blood volume may increase, with consequent hypertension. Renal disease with poor renal glomerular perfusion may result in increased renin levels. Angiotensin and aldosterone levels will then increase, with consequent vasoconstriction, sodium retention, and elevated blood pressure.

3) **Cardiac disease** may significantly impair the heart's ability to pump blood. Thus, peripheral tissues, including the kidney, will be poorly perfused, with inadequate elimination of ingested water and salt. Increased plasma volume and increased capillary blood pressure may result, leading to leakage of fluid into the interstitial spaces (**edema**).

4) Destructive tumors in the pituitary-hypothalamic region may eliminate the ability to produce ADH. In the absence of ADH, the patient may urinate 20 liters per day (a condition call **diabetes insipidus**). This will dehydrate the patient, unless the patient compensates by imbibing an equal amount of water. Conversely, with **excess production of ADH** (e.g. in the syndrome of inappropriate ADH secretion, which occurs especially with certain pulmonary and brain tumors), the blood volume increases (unless there is water restriction) and so may the blood pressure.

5) **Tumors of the adrenal medulla** (pheochromocytomas) may secrete excess **epinephrine and norep-**inephrine, thereby raising the blood pressure, as will adrenal cortical tumors that produce aldosterone (**primary hyperaldosteronism**). Excess aldosterone may also arise secondary to excess renin production (**secondary hyperaldosteronism**), which may occur with renin-producing juxtaglomerular cell tumors or, more commonly, with renal artery stenosis and many kinds of renal disorders. Plasma renin, while high in secondary hyperaldosteronism, is low in primary hyperaldosteronism, because elevated aldosterone normally decreases renin secretion by negative feedback.

6) The greater the rigidity of the arterial wall, as in **arteriosclerosis**, the greater the rise in systolic blood pressure. Arteriosclerotic damage also **decreases the normal endothelial cell nitric oxide**, and nitric oxide then is not available to perform its normal vasodilatory function.

7) When one **stands perfectly still**, the **venous pump** (the tendency to move the venous blood through skeletal muscle contraction) does not work efficiently in the lower extremities. Blood pools in the lower extremities, reducing the blood volume and pressure in the upper extremities. The higher resulting pressure in the veins in the legs increases the capillary pressure in the lower extremity veins, resulting in leakage of fluid into the extracellular space and edema of the lower extremities with reduction of blood volume, and hence blood pressure.

8) **Idiopathic hypertension.** Even when all control mechanisms are operating, they may not be so finely tuned quantitatively. The body may react to rises in blood pressure, but without sufficient control to achieve a normal baseline blood pressure. Such individuals may have normal laboratory tests for electrolyte balance and renal and cardiac function, but still have hypertension. **Vascular reactivity** refers to the degree of sensitivity to sympathetic stimulation of the smooth muscle in the vascular wall. Vascular reactivity may be increased in certain families who have an inherited tendency toward hypertension.

Treatment Of High and Low Blood Pressure

We have seen that the major factors involved in pressure regulation are fluid volume, vascular resistance, and cardiac output. It stands to reason that the major efforts to control hypertension involve:

1) **Reduction of plasma volume**, e.g. through salt restriction and **diuretics**, drugs that increase water excretion.

a) **Loop diuretics** (e.g. furosemide) and **thiazide diuretics** (e.g. hydrochlorothiazide) interfere with the active transport of sodium chloride, particularly in the ascending limb of Henle and the distal convoluted tubule (see Fig. 2-11, further explained in Chapter 3). Thus, sodium remains in the tubular lumen along with water; other molecules remain too, for osmotic reasons, as the excess water prevents them from passively leaving the lumen along a concentration gradient. Therefore, not only water but sodium, chloride, potassium, and other molecules are excreted in the urine.

b) **Osmotic diuretics,** such as mannitol, filter freely at the glomerulus but are not reabsorbed. Their osmotic effect keeps water and other molecules in the tubular lumen for excretion.

c) **Aldosterone antagonists**, such as **spironolactone**, interfere with the ability of aldosterone to promote sodium reabsorption and potassium secretion. Thus, sodium is excreted along with water, whereas potassium is retained. Such potassium sparing contrasts with the potassium loss that accompanies thiazide-type diuretics.

d) **Carbonic anhydrase inhibitors** (see Figs. 2-11 and 3-3) inhibit the reaction of $CO_2 + H_2O \rightarrow H^+ + HCO_3^-$, thereby inhibiting H^+ secretion in the proximal tubule, and decreasing the absorption of HCO_3^- and associated Na^+ ions.

In general, whenever sodium excretion increases, water excretion also increases, and plasma volume decreases. Water follows sodium into the urine. However, it is not always true that increased water excretion is accompanied by increased sodium excretion. It is possible for urine to increase significantly in volume while containing no significant sodium. This is because sodium reabsorption still continues beyond the loop of Henle even when ADH secretion is low. With low ADH, the permeability of the collecting ducts to water is extremely small and little can be reabsorbed despite the active reabsorption of sodium. The water then exits as a dilute urine without significant accompanying sodium.

2) **Promotion of vasodilation** to reduce peripheral resistance, as follows:

a) Medications that inhibit the sympathetic nervous system **centrally.** Stimulation of alpha-2 receptors on central sympathetic neurons inhibits sympathetic discharge. Hence, medications that stimulate alpha-2 receptors (**alpha-2 agonists**) will decrease blood pressure.

b) Medications that inhibit transmission from **peripheral** sympathetic neurons to vascular smooth muscle cells. This can be done by

i) Medications that block norepinephrine release from presynaptic sympathetic neurons.

ii) **Alpha-1 antagonists**, drugs that are **antagonistic** to sympathetic alpha-1 receptors on vascular smooth muscle cells (stimulation of vascular alpha-1 receptors normally causes vasoconstriction).

c) Medications that **directly vasodilate. Calcium channel blockers**, which inhibit the entry of calcium into muscle cells, cause vasodilation, because calcium is necessary for muscular contraction, including that of smooth muscle in arteriolar walls. **ACE (Angiotensin-Converting Enzyme) inhibitors** reduce blood pressure by preventing the conversion of angiotensin I to angiotensin II, which is a vasoconstrictor. Other vasodilators may act by enhancing the effect of vascular endothelial nitric oxide, a natural dilator.

3) **Reduction of cardiac output**. This may include attempts to reduce blood volume (restricting salt intake; use of diuretics) &/or the use of medications that reduce heart rate and stroke volume. Stimulation of sympathetic beta-1 receptors on heart muscle increases cardiac output. Hence, drugs that are **beta-1 antagonists** decrease cardiac output.

4) **Stress reduction** reduces the level of sympathetic activity.

5) **Weight loss** is also useful in reducing blood pressure, although the mechanism for this is still in debate.

Methods to deal with **low blood pressure** include the restoration of lost fluid volume (whether through blood or other fluids), and the use of vasoconstrictors. Medications to help restore defective cardiac functioning are also important in the control of blood pressure, whether the pressure is low or high.

Central Venous Pressure (CVP)

CVP, the pressure in the large veins, normally is close to 0 (about the same level of pressure as the right atrium). In either right or left heart failure, CVP may increase, because the heart cannot handle the blood that reaches it. CVP measurement, therefore, is a useful index of cardiac failure. The CVP can be elevated in the face of either a high or low systemic arterial pressure. Apart from cardiac pumping failure, an elevated CVP may also occur with:

1) Increased blood volume.
2) Arteriolar dilation, which allows the arterial pressure to be transmitted to the veins.

Increased CVP backs up pressure to the capillary level, where the increase in capillary hydrostatic pressure may cause water to leave the capillaries and enter the interstitial space; this results in **edema**. Edema of the extremities and liver, and engorgement of the neck veins will result from this backup in the case of right heart failure, whereas the same signs, plus pulmonary edema, may result from this backup in the case of left heart failure.

The CVP is an index of right atrial pressure, and its elevation may make us suspect cardiac failure in general, without specifying whether it is right or left heart failure. The **pulmonary wedge pressure**, in contrast, reflects left atrial pressure and helps distinguish right and left cardiac failure, as follows:

A catheter is threaded into the pulmonary artery and "wedged" up close to the pulmonary capillaries. The pressure recorded there is close to that of the left atrium. Normal mean pulmonary capillary wedge pressure is about 8 mm Hg. With left cardiac failure (or mitral valve stenosis, for example), there is backup of blood into the lungs with elevation of the pulmonary wedge pressure and CVP, and possibly pulmonary edema. In right cardiac failure, the wedge pressure is not elevated, and there is no pulmonary edema.

Pulmonary arterial pressure is lower in the superior lung fields than in the inferior fields because of gravity. This lower pressure results in decreased capillary diameter and blood flow in the superior fields, even to zero with very low pulmonary arterial pressures, as alveolar pressure collapses the capillaries. In times of oxygen need, increased cardiac output increases the pulmonary arterial pressure, which opens up collapsed capillaries and increases blood flow in all areas of the lungs.

BLOOD FLOW

Blood flow is the amount of blood that passes a particular point in the circulation per unit time. **Cardiac output** is blood flow that relates to the heart; it is the number of liters of blood pumped by the heart per minute, generally about 5–6 liters/min. This section is concerned with the factors that regulate blood flow through the heart (cardiac output) as well as the peripheral tissues.

At superficial glance, it would seem that the factors that control blood flow should be the same as the factors that govern blood pressure and blood volume, and that blood flow should vary directly with blood pressure and blood volume. For instance, if the blood pressure or blood volume were to drop drastically to zero, for instance, there would be poor blood flow. And increasing the arterial pressure and volume should increase the flow to the body tissues. However, blood flow does not always vary directly with blood pressure and blood volume. For instance:

1) Peripheral tissue blood flow may decrease with very low blood pressure, but also decrease with very high blood pressure that is based on intense arteriolar vasoconstriction.

2) Low blood volume may be associated with poor tissue blood flow, but so may high blood volume, if the heart pumps inadequately.

3) Blood flow from the pulmonary circulation through the lungs may be poor with either right or left heart failure. The poor pulmonary blood flow may be associated with an elevated pulmonary artery pressure in left heart failure but a decreased pulmonary artery pressure in right heart failure.

Hence, we need to look separately at the factors that regulate blood flow.

The main factors that influence flow from the **heart** (i.e., **cardiac output**—not the coronary circulation) are:

1) **The degree of cardiac contractility**. A more forceful cardiac contraction expels more blood (i.e., is associated with a greater **stroke volume**) per beat.
2) **The heart rate**. Increasing the heart rate increases the cardiac output.
3) **The venous return to the heart.** The heart pumps out whatever the veins send it. Therefore, factors that increase the rate of venous return will increase cardiac output. These include:
   a) **The blood volume**. Increased blood volume leads to greater venous return.
   b) **Patency of the venous system**. An obstruction in the vena caval system will decrease venous return
   c) **The degree of arteriolar dilation**. Arteriolar dilation decreases vascular resistance and allows more blood to enter the venous system and thus increases the rate of venous return to the heart.
   d) **The differential pressure** between the beginning and end of the circulation. The overall blood pressure, per se, is not a significant determinant of cardiac output. As mentioned previously, it is the **difference** in pressure between the beginning of the arterial tree and the end of the venous tree, rather than the mean blood pressure that is responsible for blood flow. The greater the difference, the greater the flow. The major determinant of cardiac output is venous return, not arterial blood pressure.
   e) **The skeletal muscle pump**. The heart is not the only muscle that pumps blood. Blood is also moved along (in one direction because of the presence of one-way valves in the veins) when there is active skeletal muscle contraction.
   f) **The respiratory pump**. With each inspiration, the negatively generated pressure draws blood into the heart through the venae cava. Expiration does not cancel this effect, because of the presence of the one-way venous valves.

Both the respiratory and skeletal muscle pumps become more active during exercise and contribute to increasing cardiac output. The type of exercise makes a difference. In **isometric** (static) exercise (muscle contraction without change in muscle length), the contracting muscle constricts the blood vessels, thereby raising peripheral resistance and blood pressure. The heart pumps against an increased load and performs more work with less output and a lower heart rate than in **isotonic** (dynamic) exercise (muscle contraction with change in muscle length), where the muscle anoxia results in peripheral vessel dilation rather than constriction.

The main factors that influence flow through the **peripheral tissues** are:

1) **Cardiac output.** Increased cardiac output increases peripheral flow. This can occur through an increase in cardiac contractility and stroke volume or an increase in heart rate.

The coronary artery circulation represents an interesting reversal of the normal logic about blood flow. In other blood vessels, blood flow increases during cardiac contraction. Blood flow, however, decreases in the coronary arteries during systole due to the compression of coronary vessels by the constricting cardiac muscle. It might therefore be supposed that sympathetic stimulation of the heart would decrease coronary blood flow, because it leads to more forceful and rapid cardiac muscle contractions. However, sympathetic innervation actually causes more dilation than constriction, because as heart rate and contractility increase, this increases the oxygen demand of the heart; the increased oxygen demand results in a local autoregulative chemical effect that dilates coronary vessels. Similarly, parasympathetic fibers indirectly cause an autoregulatory vasoconstriction because they slow the heart rate and decrease oxygen demands.

The systolic compression of coronary vessels has its greatest effect on the endocardial layer of the heart. Hence, the endocardium, particularly that of the left ventricle, is frequently the first area affected in **myocardial infarction** (heart attack).

2) **Blood volume.** Decreasing the blood volume decreases the tissue flow. With modest decreases, the heart can compensate by increasing its output. Blood volume may decrease for any of these reasons: decreased fluid intake, excess body loss of fluids, or shift of fluids in body compartments (as in internal hemorrhage or otherwise leaky blood vessels).

The capillary membrane is not freely permeable to all molecules. Proteins, for instance, tend to remain inside the capillary lumen, where they can exert a significant osmotic effect. In hypoproteinemia, or excess water loading in the face of poor renal functioning, fluid may leave the capillaries to cause swelling of the interstitial spaces (edema). In inflammation, the capillaries may leak protein, in which case both protein and accompanying fluid enter the extracellular spaces and reduce blood volume.

3) **The degree of vessel dilation.** Blood pressure decreases with vascular dilation, whereas blood flow increases. The greater the resistance to flow within the blood vessel, as by vasoconstriction, the lesser the flow. Turbulent flow, as may occur with irregularities in the blood vessel wall secondary to arteriosclerosis, also increases the resistance and thus decreases the blood flow.

The **Poiseuille equation** states that:

$$\text{Flow} = (\text{Pressure difference})\,\pi r^4/8Ln \text{ where}$$

r = inside radius of the vessel
L = length of the vessel
n = fluid viscosity

An important point about this equation is the fourth power of the radius, which indicates that a large change in flow occurs for any change in vessel diameter.

The state of blood vessel dilation is partially under control of the sympathetic nervous system. In the case of the skin, there is a further modifying factor—heat. The hypothalamus responds to cold through a temperature-controlling mechanism which generates sympathetic output that constricts skin blood vessels, thereby conserving heat. Excess heat is released through the skin by vasodilation secondary to sympathetic inhibition. (Parasympathetic innervation of blood vessels is insignificant.) Interestingly, at the start of exercise, blood vessels in the skin may vasoconstrict, as part of the sympathetic diversion of blood to other body areas. With continuing exercise, the body temperature rises and skin vasodilation may then occur as a heat-releasing mechanism.

4) **Viscosity of blood.** With increased viscosity, friction retards flow through blood vessels. Hematocrit (the percentage of a volume of blood that consists of cells) is the major determination of viscosity, although plasma proteins also play a role.

5) **The degree of vascularization of the tissues.** Increased vascularization of the tissues occurs as a long-range reaction to inadequate blood flow, due especially to lack of oxygen. The greater the vascularization, the greater the blood flow.

6) **Standing versus lying down.** Standing for prolonged periods causes venous pooling in the lower extremities, with decreased available blood volume and decreased general body tissue perfusion. The situation is particularly significant when venous dilation is

enough to interfere with the normal valve function of the veins, which normally help ensure that backflow in the veins does not occur.

As important as blood flow is to supplying nutrients to the tissues, it is important to note that the actual amount of nutrient that can be utilized by the tissues depends also on:

1) The concentration of nutrient in the blood.
2) The amount of available capillary surface area for diffusion (enhanced blood flow is of little use in a pathological arterial-venous shunt that bypasses capillaries).
3) The distance of diffusion from the capillary to the tissues For example, antibiotics may not be able to reach the central core of an abscess. Hence, the surgeon frequently must drain an abscess to achieve proper healing.
4) The permeability of the capillary wall (the capillary wall in the brain is impermeable to many substances that can diffuse through in other body areas. Hence, the term **blood brain barrier**). In general, lipid-soluble substances, including O_2 and CO_2, pass easily through capillary cell walls. Small ions, such as Na^+ and K^+ pass less easily, but still pass more easily than one would expect, possibly because they may pass through water-filled pores that transcend the capillary wall. Proteins are generally too large to pass through capillary walls. In cases where they do, the lymphatic system provides a way of returning them to the general circulation.

The **Fick principle** quantitates the amount of nutrient that is utilized by the tissues, starting with the premise that:

$$X' = Q'[X]$$

X' = the rate of transport of nutrient X (mass/time) along the vessel
Q' = the blood flow rate
$[X]$ = the blood concentration of X

The Fick principle extends this to simply state that the rate of utilization of the nutrient by the tissue = (the rate of transport of the nutrient to the tissue) minus (the rate of transport of the nutrient away from the tissue). The formula for this is shown as:

$$X'_{tc} = Q'X_a - Q'X_v = Q'(X_a - X_v) \text{ where:}$$

X'_{tc} = the net rate of transcapillary transport of nutrient X (i.e., the rate of utilization of the nutrient by the tissue)
Q' = the blood flow rate
X_a = the arterial concentration of the nutrient
X_v = the venous concentration of the nutrient

The Fick principle may be used to calculate the cardiac output by considering the rate of utilization of oxygen by the body as a whole. If X_a is the arterial concentration of O_2 (measured in arterial blood) and X_v is the venous concentration of O_2 (measured at the opposite end of the circulation via a catheter in the right ventricle or pulmonary artery) and X'_{tc} is the rate of utilization of oxygen by the body, then the blood flow rate through the body (cardiac output) or Q' equals $X'_{tc}/(X_a - X_v)$. For instance, if the patient utilizes 200ml of oxygen per minute and X_a = 200ml O_2/liter and X_v = 150ml O_2/liter, then Q' = 200ml/min divided by (50ml/liter) = 4 liters/min of cardiac output.

A Seeming Paradox

In profound blood loss, the blood pressure drops, and the tissues are not perfused well. Shouldn't it damage the tissues even further if the body attempts to raise blood pressure through vasoconstriction, which in itself would further decrease the perfusion? In answer:

1) It is important to realize that much of the vasoconstrictive response involves the veins rather than the arterioles, thereby allowing previously pooled blood to participate in the circulation, without damaging tissue perfusion.
2) Sympathetic innervation has relatively little effect on the coronary and cerebral arterioles, which is fortunate, as these areas in particular require adequate perfusion. In addition, epinephrine, which is released by the adrenal medulla in states of circulatory shock, has a significant vasodilator effect, as it acts on the beta-2 receptors in the blood vessels of cardiac and skeletal muscle.

The reason why some vessels constrict and some vasodilate in shock has partly to do with the distribution, on the blood vessels of the various organs, of vasodilatory versus vasoconstrictive receptors, which react oppositely to circulating epinephrine. In addition, it is important to note that sympathetic innervation and local biochemical (autoregulatory) control mechanisms both influence the state of vascular constriction, and the blood vessels of some organs have a predominantly sympathetic nerve innervation, whereas others function predominantly through autoregulatory factors. The organs with predominantly sympathetic innervation will demonstrate vasoconstriction during a state of shock, because the sympathetic nervous system is stimulated. The ones with predominantly autoregulatory control will exhibit vasodilation during shock, because the anoxia triggers local vasodilatory autoregulatory mechanisms. The heart, brain, and skeletal muscle blood vessels exhibit a predominantly autoregulatory mechanism. Thus blood flow to these areas is preserved, or even enhanced, during states of shock.

Other organs, including the digestive tract, liver, skin, and kidney have a predominantly sympathetic nerve input. Blood diverts from these organs during shock to help preserve blood pressure. This is not always good, because renal and hepatic failure can result from such shock, in which the kidney and liver circulations are sacrificed for the common good. The relatively weak effect of the sympathetic system on cerebral arterial contractility may be a good reason why the operation of sympathectomy (cutting the sympathetic nerves to the head in an effort to promote vasodilation and correct cerebrovascular insufficiency) has not been considered very successful. On the other hand, much greater success has been obtained with lumbar sympathectomy aimed at increasing circulation to the lower extremities.

3) Sympathetic stimulation increases cardiac contractility and output, thus helping to relieve the perfusion problem.

4) Although arteriolar constriction is partly balanced by an autoregulatory effect, the body, nonetheless, does appear to prefer maintaining blood pressure over maintaining tissue perfusion when there is blood volume loss. Hence, patients with hemorrhagic shock tend to have cool skin (reflecting vasoconstriction), rather than warm skin (which would occur in vasodilation).

Shock

Shock means a lot of confusing things. It could mean something that happens to you when you stick your finger into an electric socket; an emotional reaction to some sudden striking news; spinal shock in which there are loss of reflexes and other functions secondary to spinal cord injury; hypoglycemic shock in which there is decreased cerebral functioning secondary to low blood glucose levels. Usually, though, shock refers to a **general failure of the circulation** either due to fluid loss or inefficiency of the circulatory blood flow control mechanisms, resulting in tissue damage. Shock is generally characterized by hypotension, cold skin, and, often, tachycardia. Examples of **circulatory shock** (shock that originates in the circulation) include:

1) **Cardiac shock**. Circulation (cardiac output) decreases because of heart malfunction.

2) **Decreased blood volume** (e.g. hemorrhage). Also included is excessive venous dilation and blood pooling, in which the total blood volume may be normal but the effective volume is decreased.

3) **Venous or arterial obstruction**, including obstruction of the pulmonary circulation in pulmonary embolus, or circulation through the heart in cardiac

tamponade (cardiac compression from pericardial fluid effusion or hemorrhage).

4) In **anaphylactic shock**, there is release of a histamine-like chemical that results in venous and arteriolar dilation, as well as fluid loss into the interstitial spaces, due to increased capillary permeability.

5) In **adrenocortical shock,** there is failure of the adrenal cortex to produce mineralocorticoids, particularly aldosterone, leading to decreased fluid volume through loss of sodium and water.

6) In **heat stroke,** circulatory shock occurs from loss of fluids while sweating. Also the heat itself damages the central nervous system. The patient is dizzy, and may lose consciousness.

7) In **septic shock,** there is high fever with vasodilation, particularly in damaged tissues affected by bacterial toxins.

Although circulatory shock often is accompanied by decreased blood pressure, the pressure commonly is normal, as the body attempts to compensate for the shock through intense vasoconstriction. Or the person may have greatly decreased blood pressure and not be in shock when vasodilation opens up peripheral arterioles to allow tissue perfusion.

Treatment of circulatory shock includes:

1) Placing the patient in the **supine position**, with legs elevated to improve cerebral blood flow.

2) **Oxygen**, to partially compensate for circulatory failure.

3) **Correction of the underlying cause**: fluid replacement in cases of volume loss; treatment of cardiac arrhythmias; steroids in adrenocortical and anaphylactic shock; correction of venous or arterial obstruction, including anticoagulants in pulmonary embolus; antibiotics and (presently experimental) administration of monoclonal antibodies to bacterial endotoxin, in septic shock.

Vasoconstrictors may help when other measures, such as fluid replacement, are ineffective. Vasoconstrictors, though, do not correct the underlying cause of shock and may have adverse effects. Remember that vasoconstrictors, while increasing blood pressure, also decrease peripheral circulation, including that to the kidneys and liver, and may contribute to renal and hepatic failure.

The central venous pressure (CVP) can help determine the need for fluid replacement. Normal CVP is about 5–8 cm of water. A low CVP generally suggests the need for fluid replacement, whereas a CVP >15 generally suggests excess volume expansion. The CVP, though, is not always an accurate reflection of fluid need, since things other than blood volume can affect it (e.g. the CVP may be elevated with obstruction from cardiac tamponade).

Pulmonary capillary wedge pressure (PCWP) measurement is a more reliable guide to fluid need. A (**Swan-Ganz**) catheter tip is wedged into the pulmonary artery against the pulmonary capillaries. A PCWP >14 suggests that pulmonary edema may be imminent and that increasing the fluid volume may be hazardous.

CHAPTER 3.   ELECTROLYTES AND ACID-BASE METABOLISM

Electrolytes are the ionic components of the body fluids, the most notable being sodium (Na^+), potassium (K^+), chloride (Cl^-), bicarbonate (HCO_3^-), hydrogen (H^+), calcium (Ca^{++}), and phosphate (PO_4^{-3}). The precise concentrations of these electrolytes are important to body functioning, to maintain fluid osmolality and volume (sodium!), or to directly participate in body functions that require particular ions or precise pH.

Many diseases can change electrolyte concentrations. In order to understand this, one must first consider the factors that maintain normal electrolyte balance:

The kidney, unlike popular portrayals, is more than just a toilet that flushes out waste products. Its one million nephrons play a powerful role in maintaining the proper balance of numerous molecules vital to the body, such as sodium, potassium, bicarbonate, chloride, H^+, glucose, etc. The kidney is also important in the excretion of many kinds of foreign molecules, including many drugs (the liver also eliminates many drugs). It does these things through **filtration**, **reabsorption**, **secretion**, and **synthesis**:

1) **Filtration.** Filtration of molecules occurs through the **glomerular membrane.**

Fig. 3-1. The glomerular membrane contains three layers:

   a) the **capillary endothelium** of the glomerulus.

   b) the **inner wall of Bowman's capsule** (sort of like the wall of a balloon that has been punched in by a fist and which is contacting the fingers). This layer contains "**podocyte**" cells.

   c) a non-cellular glomerular **basement membrane**, which lies between the capillary endothelium and podocyte layers. (The glomerulus (Figs. 2-8, 2-9) also contains **mesangial cells.** These have contractile properties (partly stimulated by catecholamines and angiotensin II; inhibited by atrial natriuretic factor). When mesangial cells contract or relax, this respectively reduces or increases the surface area of the glomerulus, thereby altering the capacity for glomerular filtration.

The outer and inner layers of the glomerular membrane leak, since the cells do not tightly adhere to one

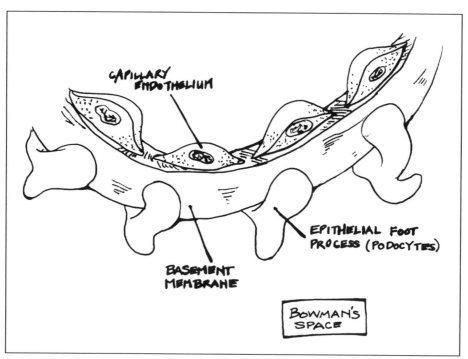

Figure 3-1

another; slit-like spaces between the cells allow the passage of small molecules. Most of the resistance to the passage of large molecules, especially to proteins, lies in the basement membrane. In addition to spatial considerations, ionic charge relationships within the glomerular membrane render it particularly difficult for large negatively charged particles to pass through (most proteins are negatively charged). The basement membrane is like a sieve that contains negative charges within its holes. Whereas large, negatively charged particles have a hard time getting through, small negatively charged particles do filter through.

2) **Reabsorption.** Once within the renal tubule lumen, molecules can be excreted or **reabsorbed,** depending on body need. Molecules that are nonpolar are reabsorbed more easily through the renal tubular membrane. Thus, if one wishes to increase the excretion of a drug that is a weak acid (e.g. aspirin overdose), it may help to alkalinize the urine. This will drive to the left the reaction:

$$H^+ + DRUG^- \leftrightarrow HDRUG$$

The more polar form of the drug produced by this reaction will then be excreted. Alternatively, one could acidify the urine to cause more of a weak acid medication to be reabsorbed.

Reabsorption of various molecules can be affected by introducing drugs that specifically block transport through the tubular epithelium. Thiazide diuretics, for instance, block the reabsorption of sodium in the distal convoluted tubule; sodium is then excreted along with water, which normally, for osmotic reasons, follows sodium passively. Probenecid inhibits the tubular **reabsorption** of urate and is used in the treatment of hyperuricemia in gout. Probenecid also inhibits the tubular **secretion** of penicillin and is used to maintain plasma levels of penicillin.

At this point, review Fig. 1-3 (mechanisms of transport across cell membranes) and Fig. 2-11 (sites of tubular absorption and secretion of key molecules).

Fig. 3-2. Reabsorption of sodium in the renal tubule. Sodium is actively transported from the renal tubular cell into the interstitial fluid and peritubular capillaries, a process that occurs throughout the length of the renal tubule. This depletes the concentration of intracellular sodium in the renal tubule cells, leading to passive diffusion of sodium from the renal tubular lumen into the tubular cell. This passive diffusion is a key driving force for much of the secondary active transport reabsorption from the renal tubular lumen of other molecules that accompany sodium via carrier molecules.

About 65% of filtered Na^+ and H_2O is reabsorbed in the proximal tubule. In addition, the proximal tubule is particularly important in the reabsorption of bicarbonate and many organic substances (e.g. glucose, amino acids, lactate, water soluble vitamins, ketones, various Krebs cycle products, etc.). These organic molecules, through secondary active transport (cotransport variety) with sodium, can move uphill against their electrochemical gradients and be almost totally reabsorbed (unless the concentration of the molecules to be absorbed is excessively high, in which case they will be excreted in the urine). Different **carrier proteins** are important in the transportation of certain groups of these organic molecules during reabsorption. The kinds of carrier molecules differ in various areas of the renal tubule. Thus, as Fig. 2-11 shows, different kinds of molecules are reabsorbed (or secreted) in different areas of the tubule, depending on which carrier molecule is present.

For instance, one particular carrier protein carries arginine, lysine, and ornithine. Another carries aspartate and glutamate. Various diseases of amino acid transport may selectively affect the reabsorption of one or more amino acids. For instance, in classic **cystinuria** there is a defect in the transport of cystine, lysine, arginine, and ornithine in the proximal renal tubule and jejunal mucosa. In **Hartnup disease**, there is a defect in the reabsorption of neutral amino acids. Other diseases, characteristically hereditary, may affect the transport of other amino acids, hexoses, urate, and various anions and cations in the renal tubule and small intestine. Some diseases may affect reabsorption, whereas others may affect secretion. For example, in **renal tubular acidosis**, H^+ cannot be properly secreted by the renal tubule. Sodium (Na^+) then is reabsorbed along with chloride (Cl^-) rather than through exchange with H^+, and a hyperchloremic acidosis develops.

Reabsorption occurs partly because the hydraulic pressure in the peritubular capillaries is very low, due to the passage of blood through the glomeruli. Also, the osmolality in the peritubular capillaries is relatively high since proteins do not filter at the glomerular level.

3) **Secretion.** Molecules that do not filter through the glomerulus pass on into the efferent renal arteriole to the peritubular capillaries, which surround the renal tubules. There, the molecules may be secreted into the tubular lumen, from which they are then excreted or reabsorbed. Some molecules are neither filtered nor secreted significantly (e.g. albumin), whereas others may be both filtered and secreted (e.g. potassium). The degree of reabsorption or secretion of a particular mole-

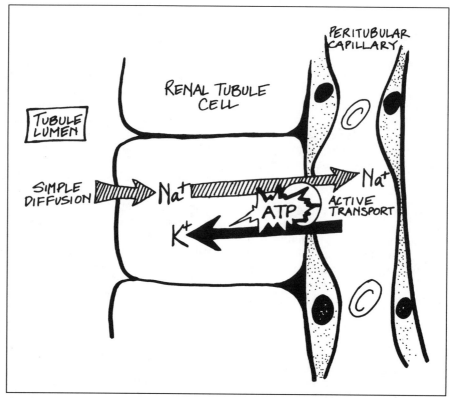

Figure 3-2

cule may be linked to the degree of reabsorption or secretion of other molecules.

4) Apart from excretion and reabsorption, the kidney also **synthesizes** various molecules, including renin, vitamin D, prostaglandins, kinins, glucose, bicarbonate, ammonia (a byproduct of amino acid metabolism that may be secreted and excreted by the kidney), and **erythropoetin**, which stimulates red cell production. Patients with renal disease may have a concurrent anemia secondary to reduced erythropoetin synthesis.

What Regulates the Amount Of Body Sodium?

Sodium is the most abundant extracellular cation (positive ion). It influences the degree of water retention in the body and is an important participant in the control of acid-base balance. Deficiency may result in neuromuscular dysfunction. Excess may result in hypertension and fluid retention. Sodium ingestion and excretion control the **total amount** of plasma sodium. The **concentration** of plasma sodium depends on the degree of its dilution with water. Factors affecting the amount and concentration of sodium include:

1) **Ingestion of sodium.** If sodium concentration is high, this affects the hypothalamus, resulting in "thirst" and imbibing of water to restore the normal concentration. Sodium intake is largely a matter of dietary habit, although, somehow, many animals also seem to know when they are salt depleted and develop a "salt hunger."

2) **Excretion of sodium**. The degree of sodium output depends partly on the plasma sodium concentration itself. If there is a low plasma sodium concentration to begin with, less sodium will get filtered and less excreted, Moreover, aldosterone, ANF, and ADH directly or indirectly influence sodium reabsorption and excretion.

Sodium filters freely through the glomerular membrane. Almost all sodium excretion occurs through the kidney. A very small amount occurs in sweat and feces, but nonrenal means of excretion may become significant with vomiting, excess sweating, diarrhea, hemorrhage, and burns. About 65% of filtered sodium and water are reabsorbed at the level of the proximal tubule; fine tuning of sodium reabsorption occurs distally, particularly in the cortical collecting duct under the influence of aldosterone.

The **amount** of sodium reabsorption in the proximal tubule remains about the same regardless of changes in glomerular filtration rate (GFR). That is, decreased GFR results in decreased filtered sodium and thus decreased reabsorption of sodium and water, whereas increased GFR results in increased reabsorption. This phenomenon (called **glomerulo-tubular balance**) helps to maintain the levels of sodium and water in the body. Part of the mechanism involves the simple point that increased GFR results in increased delivery of sodium to the tubules, and hence greater reabsorption, but the mechanism is more complex.

Glomerulo-tubular balance should not be confused with **tubuloglomerular feedback**, another autoregulatory mechanism that also guards against the effects of changes in GFR. In tubulo-glomerular feedback, an increased GFR is reflected in an increase in fluid flow through the renal tubules and past the macula densa. The macula densa senses this and feeds back a local chemical influence that constricts the afferent arterioles, thereby decreasing the GFR.

Thus, G-T balance (what the glomerulus gives to the tubules) guards against an increased GFR by increasing sodium reabsorption. T-G feedback (the information that the tubules feed back to the glomerulus) guards against an increased GFR by decreasing GFR.

Water filtration follows sodium passively, so the actual concentration of sodium in the tubular fluid does not change significantly on filtration through the glomerulus. Most sodium ends up reabsorbed, because active transport is involved in the reabsorption process, and the sodium is reabsorbed against an electrochemical gradient (Fig. 3-2). Note that water, but not sodium reabsorption occurs in the descending loop of Henle (imagine a waterfall descending and splashing out the descending loop), whereas sodium reabsorption, but not water reabsorption occurs in the ascending loop of Henle (Fig. 2-11). This ensures that the interstitium outside the ascending limb is hyperosmolar. This is important, because, as tubular fluid continues beyond the ascending limb of the loop and into the collecting tubule, where water can leave the tubule, water exits into the body circulation, thereby reducing the volume of urine. As this reduced volume continues down the collecting duct, more water passively leaves to enter the surrounding hyperosmotic interstitium, thereby enabling the urine to be concentrated, **even more so than the plasma**. The peculiar looping shape of the nephron thus has physiologic importance. It enables the formation of a very hyperosmotic interstitium in the lower levels of the loop, enabling marked concentration of the urine, when needed, while urine passes down the collecting ducts. The degree of ADH secretion helps determine whether the urine will be concentrated or dilute, because ADH increases the permeability of the collecting ducts to water, enabling water to leave the collecting ducts, resulting in a more concentrated urine.

Loop diuretics (Fig. 2-11) cause less hyponatremia than do thiazide diuretics, which act on the distal convoluted tubule, because there is still a "last chance" for sodium to be reabsorbed in the distal convoluted tubule when loop diuretics are used. Moreover, loop diuretics cause more of a diuresis than do thiazides, because by blocking sodium transport in the loop area, they prevent the interstitium in the loop area from becoming very hyperosmotic. Thus, water in the medullary collecting ducts has less osmotic tendency to enter the interstitium, and instead ends up being excreted.

About 180 liters (about 45 gallons) of water filter through the glomerular membranes of the kidney per day in the 70 kg person. Obviously, water reuptake from the renal tubules is an important aspect of fluid balance, and high urine concentration may be vital in times of water deprivation.

3) **Atrial natriuretic factor,** produced in response to dilation of the cardiac atria, as might occur with excessive blood volume, induces sodium excretion by decreasing sodium reabsorption.

4) The hypothalamus produces **antidiuretic hormone (ADH)**, the release of which is stimulated by increased plasma sodium concentration. The primary effect of ADH is promotion of reabsorption of water by the kidney, thus restoring normal serum osmolality and reducing the sodium concentration. High plasma osmolality also affects the hypothalamus to induce thirst.

Although most water in the body comes from ingested food and drink, some is metabolically generated, particularly from carbohydrate metabolism.

It is possible for the total body sodium to be elevated but the serum sodium concentration to be normal or decreased in cases where the excess sodium is diluted by an even more excessive volume of body water (e.g. in inappropriate ADH secretion; in poor renal perfusion, as in renal disease or poor cardiac output, in which water is not filtered adequately by the kidney and is retained in the body).

5) Sodium reabsorption cannot occur as an isolated event. Sodium cations need to either carry with them chloride or other anions (to avoid charge buildup in the tubular lumen) or exchange with secreted potassium or hydrogen cations.

Fig. 3-3. Mechanism of indirect absorption of bicarbonate ion in the renal tubule. HCO_3^- ions carry Na^+ ions with them when they are reabsorbed through the peritubular capillary side of the renal tubule cell. Bicarbonate anions do not pass easily through the tubular lumen side of the renal tubular cell, but can pass through indirectly as CO_2, after combining with secreted H^+ ions. In alkalosis, the blood pH is elevated. There is little H^+ to exchange with sodium in the kidney and little H^+ to facilitate bicarbonate absorption. There-

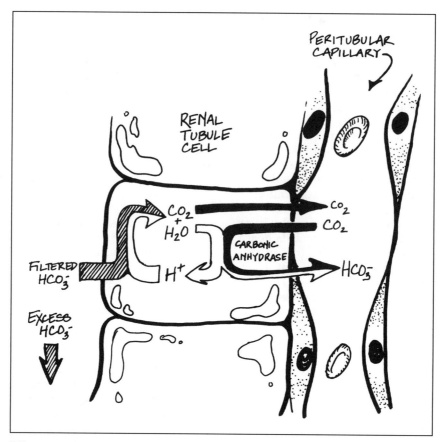

Figure 3-3

fore, reabsorption of sodium and bicarbonate decreases, while their excretion increases.

What Controls the Amount of Intra- and Extracellular Potassium?

Potassium is the main **intracellular** cation. About 98% of the body potassium is intracellular, largely the result of the sodium-potassium pump, which keeps potassium in cells. Potassium is important in all cell functioning, including myocardial depolarization and contraction. Deficiency may result in neuromuscular dysfunction; excess may cause myocardial dysfunction.

The plasma level of potassium is much lower than that of sodium. Relatively small changes in plasma potassium can have a profound effect on body functioning, and regulation must be very tight. The key factors that maintain plasma potassium levels are:

1) Dietary intake
2) Renal filtration and secretion
3) Serum pH
4) Effects of insulin and epinephrine

Regarding renal filtration and secretion, the degree of secretion of potassium into the tubular lumen partly depends on the concentration of serum potassium. Aldosterone, however, also has a very important role, because it stimulates the sodium-potassium ATPase pump and facilitates passage of sodium through the luminal membrane Na^+ channels, particularly in the cortical collecting ducts. These aldosterone effects result in the reabsorption of sodium, which is linked to the secretion of potassium into the renal tubular lumen for excretion. Aldosterone also increases the permeability of the tubular membrane to potassium. Aldosterone production increases with low blood pressure and low plasma sodium. Another stimulus to aldosterone production is a high plasma level of potassium, which directly stimulates adrenal cortical cells to produce aldosterone.

Fig. 3-4. The plasma potassium concentration also changes with the serum pH. If pH decreases (the $[H^+]$ increases), H^+ tends to enter the body's cells in exchange for K^+, and plasma $[K^+]$ increases. When blood pH increases ($[H^+]$ decreases), H^+ tends to leave cells and enter the bloodstream, to partly compensate for the

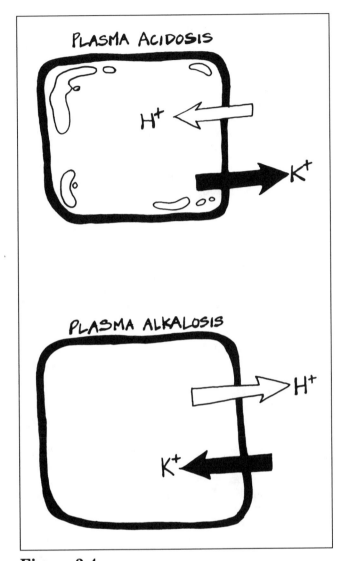

Figure 3-4

into muscle cells. Elevated plasma potassium stimulates **aldosterone** secretion, as a means of decreasing the elevated potassium. Aldosterone reduces elevated potassium levels not only through increased renal excretion of potassium but also through increased entry of potassium into cells.

Those diuretics that prevent water reuptake at the renal tubular level also prevent the uptake of sodium and potassium, because the latter, for osmotic reasons, will tend to maintain their concentrations in the increased amount of tubular water. Thus both sodium and potassium are excreted when such diuretics are used. In contrast, aldosterone inhibitors, by inhibiting aldo-sterone's effect, prevent the reuptake of sodium while preventing the secretion and subsequent excretion of potassium. The sodium that remains in the renal tubule has an osmotic effect in holding onto water. Thus, increased excretion of water and sodium, but not potassium, occur with the use of aldosterone inhibitors.

Note that aldosterone stimulates potassium secretion largely in the cortical end of the collecting duct and is not very active in the more distal medullary end of the collecting duct. ADH on the other hand acts largely on the medullary end of the collecting duct. Therefore, changes in water flow that accompany changes in ADH level do not significantly affect potassium excretion.

A conflict: What happens if both plasma potassium and extracellular volume decrease at once (e.g., in diarrhea)? One would expect the low potassium to cause a decrease in aldosterone production, with subsequent potassium retention, but the low volume should increase aldosterone production and potassium excretion. The final result may depend on the degree of potassium versus extracellular volume depletion. There may not be much net change in the amount of plasma potassium.

Primary and secondary hyperaldosteronism affect potassium levels differently. In **primary hyperaldosteronism**, plasma potassium levels drop, because aldosterone stimulates potassium secretion in the distal tubule. In **secondary hyperaldosteronism** (e.g. secondary to increased renin production from reduced GFR), potassium loss may be minimal according to the following reasoning: Low GFR means low fluid flow rate through the renal tubules; low fluid flow rate results in greater time for (sodium and) water reabsorption, and a greater concentration of potassium in the tubular fluid; increased potassium concentration in the tubular fluid decreases the gradient for potassium secretion into the tubular fluid.

alkalosis. In exchange for the H^+, K^+ enters the cells and results in a decreased plasma $[K^+]$ (**hypokalemic alkalosis**). In addition, alkalosis itself tends to enhance renal potassium secretion (with subsequent excretion) in place of H^+ secretion. Such K^+ secretion contributes to a hypokalemia. Some forms of acidosis reduce potassium secretion and excretion.

Insulin, epinephrine, and aldosterone stimulate the entry of potassium into cells. A diabetic patient may become hypokalemic with overvigorous treatment with **insulin**, so potassium levels must be watched during acute treatment of diabetic acidosis with insulin. Potassium leaves muscle cells during exercise. **Epinephrine**, also released during exercise, helps reverse this outflow, increasing potassium entry particularly

What Controls Body Levels of Chloride?

Chloride is an important anion (negative ion) in the maintenance of fluid and electrolyte balance and is an important component of gastric juice.

1) Chloride concentration generally reciprocally follows changes in bicarbonate ion, since some anion is necessary to fill in the gaps of altered bicarbonate concentration, and chloride is the most common extracellular anion. Processes that decrease (or increase) plasma bicarbonate concentration tend to increase (or decrease) plasma chloride concentration. Partly this occurs with renal exchange mechanisms. It may also occur through the **chloride shift** of hemoglobin: When CO_2 enters the red blood cell in the peripheral tissues, it rapidly changes to H^+ and $HCO3^-$ under the influence of carbonic anhydrase. The H^+ combines with hemoglobin, but bicarbonate leaves the cell in exchange for chloride. Within the lung, the chloride shifts out of the red cell (when O_2 combines with hemoglobin and H^+ is released to combine with HCO_3^- and form CO_2 for exhalation).

The body may compensate for acidosis by reabsorbing more bicarbonate (in association with sodium). The more bicarbonate that is reabsorbed with sodium, the less chloride that can be reabsorbed with sodium, for reasons of ionic balance. Thus, acidosis favors sodium and bicarbonate reabsorption and chloride excretion (hypochloremia)—except in the special condition of **hyperchloremic acidosis,** where there is a defect in the renal tubule's ability to secrete H^+. In that case, since H^+ cannot get through the tubular epithelium to neutralize intratubular HCO_3^-, HCO_3^- is not reabsorbed, and Cl^- gets reabsorbed in preference to HCO_3^-.

2) Chloride, apart from exchanging for bicarbonate, also tends to follow sodium. Processes that increase or decrease sodium ion levels tend to correspondingly increase or decrease chloride levels.

What Controls PH?

The pH is the concentration of hydrogen ions, according to the formula

$$pH = \log 1/[H^+]$$

The higher the hydrogen ion concentration, the greater the acidity and the lower the pH. Normal arterial pH is 7.4, but body pH may vary from <3 in gastric secretion to >8 in pancreatic secretion. Hydrogen ions are added to or removed from the body in several ways:

1) **Diet**. This is a minor factor and may vary from a relatively acidic input, as in high protein diets, to a relatively alkaline input in mainly vegetarian diets.
2) **Metabolic production of CO_2 by the body**.

$$CO_2 + H_2O \leftrightarrow HCO_3^- + H^+$$

In the above equation, CO_2 may be considered a weak acid which is constantly being generated by the body. Being a gas, CO_2 is dealt with through the lungs. Other kinds of acids (such as lactic, phosphoric, and sulfuric acids, and ketone bodies) cannot be released by respiration. The kidney deals with these. Raw H^+ does not filter significantly through the glomeruli because most of it is bound to proteins, rather than floating free in the plasma. However, binding to plasma proteins usually does not impair tubular H^+ secretion. H^+ is secreted by the renal tubules through CO_2, which passes much more readily than H^+ from the bloodstream into the renal tubule cells.

3) **Regulation through the gastrointestinal tract**. H^+ ions are lost during vomiting, whereas HCO_3^- ions are lost (the equivalent of a gain in H^+) in diarrhea.
4) **The influence of other electrolytes** on hydrogen ion concentration. **Chloride depletion** and K^+ **depletion**, when marked, stimulate H^+ secretion into the renal tubule lumen, resulting in a metabolic alkalosis. One reason this happens is that intraluminal sodium, in those conditions, exchanges in the renal tubule for H^+ because the sodium cannot exchange for potassium or be accompanied by chloride during reabsorption.

Sodium depletion also causes H^+ loss. Sodium depletion results not only in heightened sodium reabsorption, but also in increased H^+ secretion into the renal tubules, since H^+ exchanges for sodium during the increased sodium reabsorption. There is also a stimulation of bicarbonate reabsorption with the sodium. Salt depletion also stimulates aldosterone secretion, which has a stimulatory effect on H^+ secretion. One of the reasons for this aldosterone effect is that aldosterone stimulates potassium loss, which in turn stimulates H^+ secretion, as mentioned above. Marked metabolic alkalosis may thus occur with the combination of hyperaldosteronism and potassium depletion.

5) **Buffers**. A narrow blood pH range, centering around 7.4, is critical to normal physiologic functioning of most body tissues. The body prevents pH from straying too far from the normal through buffering systems.

The ingredients of a buffering system include a mixture of molecules that prevent the pH from changing significantly on adding acid or base. This commonly consists of the mixture of a **weak acid** and its **conjugate base**. For instance, consider the equation:

$$HB \text{ (weak acid)} \leftrightarrow H^+\text{(strong acid)} + B^- \text{ (conjugate weak base)}$$

In such a case, addition to the mixture of a strong acid does not drastically lower the pH, because the weak base partly neutralizes the added acid. The reaction moves to the left, reducing the amount of added H^+.

Similarly, adding a strong base does not drastically raise the pH. The H^+ partly neutralizes it, moving the reaction to the right to provide replacement for the H^+ that was used to neutralize the base. There are a number of buffering systems in the body:

a) **The bicarbonate buffer system.** This is the main **extracellular** buffering system and the one generally thought of in considering clinical matters of acid-base balance. (The main **intracellular** buffers are proteins and phosphates.) The weak acid and conjugate base are H_2CO_3 and HCO_3^- respectively, which interact in the general reaction:

$$H_2CO_3 \leftrightarrow H^+ + HCO_3^-$$

Because the amount of undissociated H_2CO_3 is minimal, the weak acid, for all practical purposes, may be considered to be CO_2:

$$CO_2 + H_2O \leftrightarrow H_2CO_3 \leftrightarrow H^+ + HCO_3^-$$

Thus, the addition of a strong acid (H^+) will move the reaction to the left, toward CO_2 and H_2O, rather than leaving an abundance of H^+ floating around the bloodstream. This leftward shift will blunt the effect of the added H^+, and the result will be less acidic than would otherwise be the case. Similarly, the addition of a strong base (e.g. OH^-) will move the reaction to the right, because the H^+ on the right disappears; CO_2 and H_2O combine to form H^+ and HCO_3^-, thereby replenishing some H^+ and rendering the final result less alkaline than it would otherwise be.

The buffering system is a good way of fine-tuning the pH. **However, even a good buffering system will not totally restore pH to the original state, especially when the body is faced with extreme changes in acidity and alkalinity. The body thus uses two other critical control mechanisms for pH control—that of the lungs and that of the kidneys.** These organs do this partly through regulating blood CO_2 and HCO_3^- concentrations.

The **lungs** primarily affect CO_2 concentration (CO_2 being a gas), through the exhalation of excess CO_2. Bicarbonate, not being a gas, is primarily regulated by the kidney. The lungs influence CO_2 levels through brain stem respiratory centers that respond indirectly to alterations in CO_2 levels. Increased blood CO_2 or H^+ levels stimulate the brain stem respiratory centers to increase respiration, blow off CO_2, and decrease blood acidity. Actually, the main stimulus to the brain stem neurons is H^+, but H^+ does not cross the blood-brain barrier easily. CO_2 does, and then reacts with water to produce the necessary H^+ ions, which in turn stimulate the respiratory center cells to increase respiration and blow off CO_2.

Blood O_2 levels also influence respiration. Blood O_2 commonly is inversely related to blood CO_2 levels. That is, when CO_2 increases, there commonly is a decrease in O_2. Oxygen affects the carotid and aortic bodies, which are stimulated by low O_2 levels and relay this information to the brain via cranial nerves 9 and 10 to stimulate respiration. H^+ and CO_2 levels have minimal effects on the carotid and aortic bodies in comparison with their direct effects on the brain stem.

The partial pressure of CO_2 (pCO_2) in the blood is generally used as an index of blood CO_2 concentration, because the partial pressure of a gas various directly with its concentration, and pCO_2 is more easily measured than the blood concentration of CO_2. (Similarly, blood pO_2 is used as an index of the blood oxygen concentration.)

In the kidney, bicarbonate filters freely through the glomerulus but in itself is poorly reabsorbed through the luminal membrane of the tubule cell (in comparison with chloride, which the renal tubules reabsorb well). Bicarbonate reabsorption occurs indirectly through interaction with secreted H^+ (Fig. 3-3).

The kidney deals with a low bicarbonate, acidotic state both by adding to the blood new bicarbonate that it generates in the renal tubular cell, and also by the secretion of H^+, which then is excreted. Virtually all H^+ ions that are excreted in the urine are first secreted by the renal tubule cell.

Because cell membranes are more permeable to CO_2 than they are to H^+, an elevated plasma pCO_2 is a better stimulus to H^+ excretion by the kidney than is a decreased plasma pH.

Normally the body produces more acid than base each day. Therefore, the pH of the urine is generally acidic (about 6.0), but may be basic under other circumstances, where the plasma is relatively alkalotic.

b) **The phosphate and ammonia buffers.** Urine can normally be acid or alkaline, depending on the need to excrete or preserve H^+. Excess H^+ can be neutralized and excreted by combining with phosphate or ammonia buffers:

$$H^+ + HPO_4^{-2} \text{ (conjugate weak base)} \leftrightarrow H_2PO_4^-$$
$$\text{(weak acid)}$$
$$H^+ + NH_3 \text{ (conjugate weak base)} \leftrightarrow NH_4^+ \text{ (weak acid)}$$

Fig. 3-5. Regulation of H+ excretion in the kidney by interaction with phosphate or ammonia. The phosphate buffer system is also very important in intracellular fluids (where phosphate is concentrated).

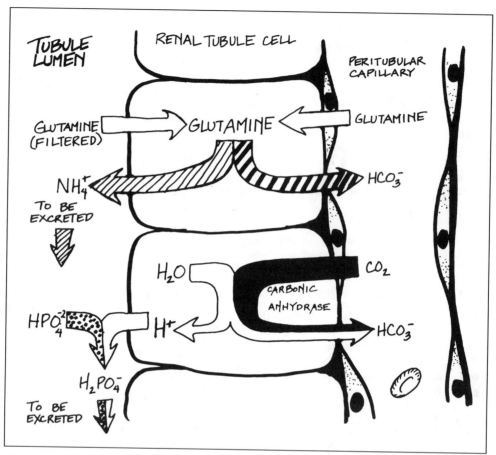

Figure 3-5

c) **The protein buffer**. H-protein and protein⁻ are the weak acid and weak conjugate base in this buffer system, which is mainly useful intracellularly:

H-protein (weak acid) $\leftrightarrow$ H⁺ + protein⁻ (conjugate weak base)

The buffering relations in the bicarbonate system are described quantitatively in the **Henderson-Hasselbach** equation:

Recalling the reaction: $CO_2 + H_2O \leftrightarrow H^+ + HCO_3^-$, the Henderson-Hasselbach equation states:

$$pH = 6.1 + \log HCO_3^-/CO_2$$

A simpler way of stating this relationship in qualitative terms is:

$$pH \propto HCO_3^-/CO_2$$

In this relationship, it may be seen that the pH will decrease with either an increase in CO_2 concentration or a decrease in HCO_3^- concentration. The buffering system helps prevent marked changes in pH. If the HCO_3^- concentration, for instance, suddenly drops, it does not cause that great a change in pH, because the CO_2 also drops (as the reaction moves to the right), while HCO_3^- is partially restored. The body tries to maintain a constant pH, so the ratio of HCO_3^- to dissolved CO_2 (carbonic acid) remains at about 20:1.

When Things Go Wrong

As we have seen, the body's buffer system, plus actions of the lungs and kidney, help maintain blood pH in the normal range. However, excesses of acid or base can significantly change pH to pathological levels. In clinical practice, blood gases and pH are measured on a sample of arterial blood.

Fig. 3-6. Changes in respiratory and metabolic acidosis and alkalosis. Consider the reaction:

$$CO_2 + H_2O \rightarrow H^+ \text{ (strong acid)} + HCO_3^- \text{ (mild base)}$$

A RESPIRATORY ACIDOSIS (uncompensated)	$\downarrow$ pH	$\dfrac{NL\ [HCO_3-]}{\uparrow[pCO_2]}$
B RESPIRATORY ACIDOSIS (compensated)	NL pH	$\dfrac{\uparrow[HCO_3-]}{\uparrow[pCO_2]}$
C METABOLIC ACIDOSIS (uncompensated)	$\downarrow$ pH	$\dfrac{\downarrow[HCO_3-]}{NL[pCO_2]}$
D METABOLIC ACIDOSIS (compensated)	NL pH	$\dfrac{\downarrow[HCO_3-]}{\downarrow[pCO_2]}$
E RESPIRATORY ALKALOSIS (uncompensated)	$\uparrow$ pH	$\dfrac{NL[HCO_3-]}{\downarrow[pCO_2]}$
F RESPIRATORY ALKALOSIS (compensated)	NL pH	$\dfrac{\downarrow[HCO_3-]}{\downarrow[pCO_2]}$
G METABOLIC ALKALOSIS (uncompensated)	$\uparrow$ pH	$\dfrac{\uparrow[HCO_3-]}{NL[pCO_2]}$
H METABOLIC ALKALOSIS (compensated)	NL pH	$\dfrac{\uparrow[HCO_3-]}{\uparrow[pCO_2]}$
I MIXED RESPIRATORY & METABOLIC ACIDOSIS	$\downarrow$ pH	$\dfrac{\downarrow[HCO_3-]}{\uparrow[pCO_2]}$
J MIXED RESPIRATORY & METABOLIC ALKALOSIS	$\uparrow$ pH	$\dfrac{\uparrow[HCO_3-]}{\downarrow[pCO_2]}$

Figure 3-6

In **respiratory acidosis**, which might occur in advanced pulmonary disease, the lungs do not adequately remove excess CO_2, and the blood becomes acidic because of CO_2 buildup (see A in Fig. 3-6).

Because the lungs are not functioning well enough to compensate for this acidity, the kidney tries to compensate by increasing its reabsorption of HCO_3^-. If the insult is not too severe, there may be compensation for the acidosis (see B in Fig. 3-6) in which case both HCO_3^- and pCO_2 will be elevated. The increased bicarbonate often is accompanied by a reciprocal decrease in chloride, as chloride typically follows an inverse relationship to bicarbonate.

Metabolic acidosis means the addition to the body of an acid, other than carbonic acid (e.g. excess apirin in-

gestion, lactic acidosis, or diabetic ketosis), or the loss of bicarbonate from the body (e.g. in severe diarrhea). HCO_3^- is markedly decreased (see C in Fig. 3-6). The respiratory centers respond to the acidosis by increasing respiration, thereby driving off CO_2, to a degree that the pCO_2 may become subnormal, and the pH approaches normal (see D in Fig. 3-6).

In **respiratory alkalosis**, which might occur with psychogenic hyperventilation, CO_2 is blown off in excess (see E in Fig. 3-6). The kidneys compensate for the alkalosis by excreting more HCO_3^- (see F in Fig. 3-6).

In **metabolic alkalosis**, there is an increase in plasma HCO_3^-. This may occur with excess ingestion of bicarbonate, with loss of stomach HCl through protracted vomiting, or with other causes. The loss of H^+ drives the reaction to the right, with an increase in bicarbonate (see G in Fig. 3-6). There is inadequate stimulation of respiratory centers because of the reduced H^+. With decreased respiratory activity, CO_2 is retained during compensation (see H in Fig. 3-6).

A reciprocal decrease in chloride commonly accompanies the increase in bicarbonate in metabolic alkalosis.

In a general way, then, the lungs try to compensate for a metabolic acidosis or alkalosis by doing their thing, changing the pCO_2; the kidneys try to compensate for a respiratory acidosis or alkalosis by doing their thing, changing the HCO_3^-. The lungs compensate by decreasing pCO_2 in metabolic acidosis and increasing pCO_2 in metabolic alkalosis. The kidneys compensate by increasing HCO_3^- in respiratory acidosis and decreasing HCO_3^- in respiratory alkalosis.

It is possible for a patient to have a mixed metabolic/respiratory acid-base problem, in which more complex HCO_3^-/pCO_2 ratios arise. For instance, in all the preceding classic examples, changes in the HCO_3^- and pCO_2 are always in the same direction; one is never elevated while the other is decreased. However, in a mixed respiratory and metabolic acidosis, the pH, of course, is decreased, and the pCO_2 may be elevated from the respiratory part, but the HCO_3^- may be decreased from the metabolic part (see I in Fig. 3-6).

Likewise, in a mixed respiratory and metabolic alkalosis, the pH, of course, is increased, and the pCO_2 may be decreased from the respiratory part, but the HCO_3^- may be increased from the metabolic part (see J in Fig. 3-6).

The arterial pO_2 may help refine the diagnosis. For instance, if the pH is increased, and both pCO_2 and HCO_3^- are decreased, one may infer a respiratory alkalosis, due to hyperventilation. However, this information does not tell us whether the hyperventilation is due to psychogenic causes or to hypoxic stimulation of hyperventilation due to pulmonary disease. A high pO_2 would suggest psychogenic hyperventilation (or overactivity of a mechanical ventilator).

The **anion gap** is a useful way of distinguishing between various kinds of acidoses:

$$\text{Anion gap} = [Na^+] - [Cl^- + HCO_3^-]$$

Sodium, chloride, and bicarbonate are the most abundant major plasma electrolytes. In order to maintain charge balance, the concentration of anions (negative ions) must equal the concentration of cations (positive ions). The normal anion gap is only 8-12 meq/L, the difference reflecting other plasma anions.

Commonly, the anion gap remains normal in an acidosis that is due to simple HCO_3^- loss (as in diarrhea and certain renal diseases) because, as a general principle, $[Cl^-]$ increases to meet the drop in HCO_3^- anions, thereby maintaining anionic balance. The anion gap may become significant, though, in various kinds of acidoses where there is an excess of certain kinds of anions (e.g., lactate in lactic acidosis; keto acids in diabetic and alcoholic ketoacidoses and starvation; phosphate, sulfate, and other organic acid ion accumulation in renal failure; salicylate poisoning in aspirin overdose; glycolate in ethylene glycol poisoning; lactate, formate and keto acids in methanol poisoning). The presence of an anionic gap provides a clue as to the underlying cause of the acidosis.

What Controls Plasma Calcium and Phosphate Levels?

Calcium is the most abundant of the body's minerals. It is an important component of bones and teeth and a participant in many metabolic processes. When bound to the receptor protein **calmodulin**, calcium helps modulate the activities of many enzymes. Calcium is important in regulation of blood clotting, neural and muscular activity, cell motility, hormone actions, and other important metabolic functions. Deficiency is associated with poor bone mineralization in rickets and osteomalacia; tetany (muscle spasm, especially in the wrists and ankles); and other neuromuscular problems. Excess causes hypercalcemia and renal stones.

Phosphate, apart from being an important component of bone, is universally important in the structure and functioning of all cells, including its presence in DNA. Deficiency is associated with rickets in children, and osteomalacia in adults. Other defects occur in the

functioning of red and white blood cells, platelets, and the liver.

Whereas calcium balance is partly controlled at the renal level, alteration of intestinal absorption of calcium is the main way of regulating calcium levels in the body. (Intestinal absorption is also the main way of controlling iron and zinc balance.)

1) **Parathyroid hormone** raises blood calcium levels. Indirectly, it promotes intestinal absorption of Ca^{++} by stimulating the activation of vitamin D in the kidney to 1,25-dihydroxycholecalciferol, which directly promotes intestinal absoption of Ca^{++}. Activation of vitamin D may also be the reason why parathyroid hormone promotes the resorption of bone, another cause of increased blood calcium.
Parathyroid hormone also increases renal tubular reabsorption of calcium (particularly in the distal renal convoluted tubule), which also increases plasma calcium levels.
2) **Vitamin D** in LARGE amounts has a similar effect as parathyroid hormone—promoting bone breakdown. But when present in only small amounts, it induces bone calcification, possible through its effect in increasing calcium uptake in the intestines and kidney.
Phosphate enters the blood with calcium when vitamin D promotes calcium absorption in the intestine, bone breakdown, and renal tubular calcium reabsorption. This could lead to dangerous levels of phosphate in the blood. To counterbalance this, parathyroid hormone has an important effect opposite to that of vitamin D. It **inhibits** renal reabsorption of phosphate, acting at the level of the proximal tubule.
Patients with renal disease may develop renal rickets through vitamin D deficiency.
3) **Calcitonin** acts the opposite of parathyroid hormone. It causes bone uptake of Ca^{++} and reduces plasma calcium levels. (Calcitonin, though, is a relatively minor influence in comparison with PT hormone and vitamin D.)
4) **pH**: Decreased pH (increased H^+) decreases calcium binding to plasma proteins, since H^+ competes for binding sites. More calcium binds to protein in alkalosis, and in alkalosis (e.g. in hyperventilation) the patient may be subject to **tetany** (single, strong, continuous muscle contractions) from the hypocalcemia.

Other Important Minerals

Magnesium is an important participant in reactions that involve ATP. Deficiency is associated with metabolic and neurologic dysfunction. Excess is associated with central nervous system toxicity.

Important trace elements include the following (in alphabetical order):

Chromium enhances the effect of insulin. Deficiency results in defective glucose metabolism. Excess occurs in chronic inhalation of chromium dust and may lead to carcinoma of the lung.

Cobalt is part of the vitamin B_{12} molecule. Excess may result in gastrointestinal distress and neurologic and cardiac dysfunction.

Copper is part of a number of enzymes, including cytochrome oxidase and lysyl oxidase (important in collagen cross-linking). Deficiency may result in anemia and mental retardation. Excess results in liver disease, various neurologic disturbances, dementia, and copper cataracts. These occur in **Wilson's disease**, in which excess copper deposits in the brain, liver, cornea, lens, and kidney.

Fluoride contributes to the hardness of bones and teeth. Deficiency is associated with dental caries. Excess is associated with stained teeth, nausea, other gastrointestinal disturbances, and tetany.

Iodide is part of the hormone thyroxine. Deficiency results in hypothyroidism. Excess results in hyperthyroidism.

Iron is an important part the hemoglobin molecule, certain enzymes, and the intracellular cytochrome system. Deficiency results in anemia. Excess results in **hemochromatosis** (abnormal iron deposits) and damage to the liver, pancreas, and other tissues.

Manganese is needed to activate a variety of enzymes, including enzymes involved in the synthesis of glycoproteins, proteoglycans and oligosaccharides. Manganese deficiency may result in underproduction of these molecules. Excess may result in Parkinson-like symptoms (shaking, slowness, stiffness, and psychosis).

Molybdenum is an important component of certain enzymes (e.g. xanthine oxidase).

Nickel may stabilize the structure of nucleic acids and cell membranes. Excess may be associated with carcinoma of the lung.

Selenium is part of the enzyme glutathione peroxidase, which, like vitamin E, acts as an antioxidant. Deficiency may result in congestive heart failure. Excess causes "garlic" breath, body odor, and skeletal muscle degeneration.

Silicon is associated with many mucopolysaccharides and may be important in the structuring of connective tissue. Excess, as may be cause by inhaling silica particles, may result in pulmonary inflammation (**silicosis**).

Zinc is a component of many enzymes, including lactate dehydrogenase and alkaline phosphatase. Deficiency is associated with poor wound healing, hypogonadism, decreased taste and smell, poor growth, and other problems. Excess is associated with vomiting from gastrointestinal irritation.

CHAPTER 4. EVALUATION OF RENAL FUNCTION

One way to measure renal function is to check the blood level of **creatinine** (which orginates from muscle creatine breakdown) or **urea** (from protein catabolism). These are waste products that normally are excreted by the kidney but accumulate in the blood in marked renal dysfunction. However, these simple lab tests are not completely accurate. Urea can be elevated for other reasons than decreased renal function, such as increased protein intake and increased tissue catabolism. Creatinine levels may differ, depending on the degree of musculature and muscular activity. Simply measuring the volume of urine output is useful but is an inadequate measure of renal function, since many factors other than renal disease can affect fluid output (e.g., the amount of fluid ingested, the blood level of ADH, and skin, GI, and respiratory fluid losses).

The **glomerular filtration rate (GFR)** is a more accurate measure of renal function. The GFR is the amount of fluid that filters through the glomerular membrane per unit of time. The GFR depends on the **filtration pressure** at the level of the glomerulus, but also on the **permeability of the glomerular membrane** and the **surface area of the glomerular membrane**. Obviously, no matter how high the filtration pressure, no fluid will filter if the glomerular membrane is not permeable or has zero surface area.

$$GFR = \text{(net filtration pressure)} \times \text{(surface area)} \times \text{(hydraulic permeability)}$$

However, it is difficult to determine net filtration pressure, surface area and hydraulic permeability. Instead, there is a different equation which incorporates entities that can easily be measured:

$GFR = UV/P$ (Imagine ultraviolet light shining on pee)

That is:

$$GFR = \text{(Urine creatinine concentration)} \times \text{(Urine vol. collected/24 hr)/(Plasma creatinine concentration)}$$

A simple derivation of the formula is as follows:

$$\text{(Mass of creatinine excreted/ time)} = \text{(Mass of creatinine filtered/ time)}$$

Note: No significant amounts of creatinine are reabsorbed or secreted. That is the reason for selecting creatinine rather than other molecules.

$$\text{(Mass of creatinine excreted/ time)} = \text{(Urine conc. of creatinine)} \times \text{(Urine vol./time)}$$

$$\text{(Mass of creatinine filtered/time)} = \textbf{(Glomerular conc.}\text{ of filtered creatinine)} \times \text{(Vol. of glomerular fluid filtered/ time)}$$

Note: The **glomerular concentration** of filtered creatinine is about the same as the **plasma concentration** of creatinine, as there is free diffusion across the glomerular membrane. Therefore:

$$\text{(Mass of creatinine filtered/time)} = \textbf{(Plasma conc. of creatinine)} \times \text{(Vol. of glomerular fluid filtered/time)} = \text{Mass of creatinine excreted/time}$$

As the volume of glomerular fluid filtered/time is the GFR, the latter equation can also be written as:

$$\text{(Mass of creatinine excreted)/time} = \text{(Plasma conc. of creatinine)} \times GFR$$

Rearranging the above equations:

$$GFR = \text{(Urine conc. of creatinine)} \times \text{(Urine vol./time)} /\text{(Plasma conc. of creatinine)}$$

or simply:

$$GFR = UV\backslash P$$

The molecule **inulin** may be used to test GFR, since creatinine does get minimally secreted (but not enough to make a big difference), whereas inulin is not secreted at all. Inulin, however, does not occur naturally and has to be continuously perfused intravenously to maintain its plasma concentration throughout the test.

The term **clearance** is somewhat different from the term GFR, even though the equation is the same:

$$\text{Clearance (of substance Y)} = \text{(Urine conc. of substance Y)} \times \text{(Urine volume collected/24 hr)/(Plasma conc. of substance Y)}$$

Clearance is the volume of plasma that is actually completely cleansed of a particular substance per unit of time for excretion of that substance in the urine. For instance, imagine the kidney as a giant nephron in which 1 drop of plasma, with its dissolved creatinine, is squeezed every 2 seconds through the mutant kidney's giant glomerular membrane cheesecloth. Imagine that all the filtered creatinine eventually gets excreted, whereas most of the filtered water in each drop gets reabsorbed in the tubules. Imagine the rest of the water being excreted, but replenished in the blood stream by ingested water. The net plasma volume remains the same. The volume of plasma, then, that is cleared (cleansed) of creatinine per second is 1 drop/2 seconds, or 0.5 drop/sec. That is also the glomerular filtration rate.

Creatinine clearance is the same as the GFR. **Glucose clearance** normally is zero, though. Glucose is totally reabsorbed from the renal tubule after it undergoes glomerular filtration; the GFR remains the same (the GFR is ALWAYS the same in a given patient, regardless of which molecule is tested), but the glucose clearance is zero, since none of the plasma ends up being cleared of glucose in the net result; the urine concentration of glucose is zero. Similarly, **albumin clearance** essentially is 0, as albumin does not filter significantly.

Consider **para-aminohippurate (PAH)**, however. This is a synthetic chemical that not only is filtered, but in addition, is secreted into the renal tubule. It is secreted so thoroughly that all the the PAH that misses being filtered and leaves via the efferent arteriole with the rest of the unfiltered plasma ends up getting secreted into the renal tubule. The numerical value for the **PAH clearance** (in volume/unit time, of course) therefore not only exceeds the GFR, but is in fact the equivalent of the total renal blood flow through the giant glomerulus. (Actually, PAH clearance is not a measure of the total renal blood flow through the kidney per se, since not all blood going to the kidney feeds the renal tubular system, but it is a measure of the **effective renal plasma flow** through the glomerulus.) In general, then:

1) The GFR is the same regardless of which substance is tested.

2) If the clearance of a substance is less than the GFR, some reabsorption of the substance is occurring, or it's not getting filtered well.

3) If the clearance of a substance exceeds the GFR, some secretion of that substance is occurring.

In practical terms, it is the GFR that one generally is interested in clinically, and measuring the creatinine clearance is a common way of assessing this. For a quick scan of the clinical situation, it usually suffices simply to obtain the plasma concentration of creatinine or urea to determine if renal function is adequate, but, as mentioned, this is not as accurate as measuring clearance.

One can quantitate the ability of the kidney to concentrate urine by calculating the **free water clearance**, which is the amount of pure water that would have to be added or subtracted from the urine to make the urine isoosmotic to plasma. That is, if the urine is less concentrated than the plasma, the free water clearance is positive, since extra water is excreted along with the excreted solute. If the urine is more concentrated than plasma, the free water clearance is negative, since relatively more water is reabsorbed.

The formula for free water clearance (C_{H2O}) is:

$$C_{H2O} = V - (U_{osmol} \times V)/P_{osmol}$$

where V is the volume of urine produced per unit of time, U_{osmol} is the urine osmolality and P_{osmol} is the plasma osmolality. If $U_{osmol} = P_{osmol}$, the free water clearance is zero. Free water clearance decreases with an increase in ADH secretion, and increases with a decrease in ADH secretion. Note that **free water clearance** is **not** the same as **water clearance**, which is the amount of water removed from the plasma per unit time.

CHAPTER 5.   EVALUATION OF CARDIAC FUNCTION

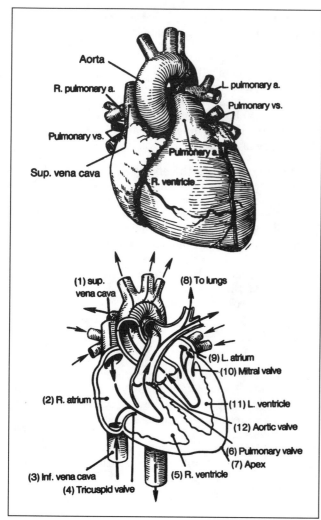

Figure 5-1

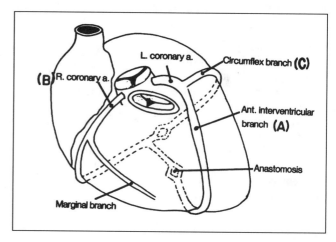

Figure 5-2

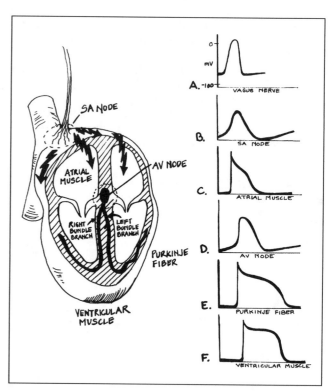

Figure 5-3

The Cardiac Cycle

Fig. 5-1. The anatomy of the heart.

Fig. 5-2. The coronary arterial circulation. A, B, and C are the most commonly occluded vessels in a myocardial infarction, in decreasing order of occurrence.

Fig. 5-3. Electrophysiologic conduction system of the heart.

The rhythmic beating of the heart originates in the modified muscle fibers of the sinoatrial (SA) node, which lies in the right atrium near the entry of the superior vena cava (Fig. 5-3). The SA node spontaneously depo-larizes from 60–100 times/min. Impulses spread rapidly from the SA node along individual atrial muscle cells to depolarize the right and left atria, which then contract to fill the right and left ventricles (**diastole**).

After a slight delay, the impulses from the atria enter the atrioventricular (AV) node. From there, impulses spread rapidly along a system of specialized conducting muscle fibers (**Purkinje fibers**) to depolarize the regular muscle cells of the ventricles, leading to ventricular contraction (**systole**). The delay at the AV node helps ensure that there is enough time for the ventricles to fill. The rapid conduction through the Purkinje fibers enables the ventricular muscle fibers to contract simultaneously, allowing a nearly synchronous and more efficient propulsion of blood from the right and left ventricles.

Although the SA and AV nodes (and the atrial and ventricular muscles themselves) have pacemaker potential, the SA node is the normal cardiac pacemaker, because it depolarizes at a faster rate than the rest of the conduction system (60–100 beats/min). The AV node spontaneously depolarizes more slowly (about 40–60 beats/min in the absence of SA node function). The ventricular musculature has a spontaneous discharge of about 20–40 times/min in the total absence of conduction system stimulation. Spontaneous discharge of the AV node and ventricular muscle, however, normally does not occur because of **capture** of the rhythm by the SA node. Thus, in the absence of an SA node, the AV node will then drive the heart beat, albeit at a slower rate than normal. In the absence of the SA and AV node functions, a slower ventricular rhythm will prevail. These backup mechanisms help ensure that the ventricles will continue beating in the presence of defects to SA and/or AV nodal discharges.

The right coronary artery supplies both the SA node (50% of the time) and AV node (90%). Sometimes the SA or AV node is supplied by branches from the left circumflex artery. Such anatomical variations are important in determining the kinds of clinical problems that arise with occlusion of a coronary artery.

An understanding of the mechanisms of electrical activity in the heart is important in the interpretation of the electrocardiogram (ECG) and in the planning of cardiac drug therapy. It will first help to review the mechanisms of maintenance of the cell membrane electric potential and triggering of the action potential. The nerve cell axon provides a classic example:

The Nerve Impulse

Like other cells in the body, the axon maintains a resting electrical membrane potential such that **the outside of the cell is more positive than the inside**.

Fig. 5-4. The Na^+/K^+ ATP pump. An ATP-driven sodium/potassium pump moves sodium out of the cell and moves potassium in. In the resting state, therefore, the concentration of sodium ions is much greater out-

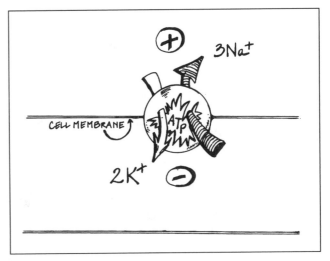

Figure 5-4

side the cell than inside, whereas the concentration of potassium is much greater inside the cell than outside.

If that were the whole story, there would be no electrical potential difference across the cell membrane, because the pump would just be exchanging one positive charge (Na^+) for another (K^+). However, there is a charge difference because:

A. The pump moves out 3 sodiums for every 2 potassiums that it pumps in.
B. Potassium leaks back outside the cell more easily than sodium leaks back in.

The above mechanisms maintain the resting membrane potential. **In addition**, there are separate voltage-dependent Na^+ and K^+ channels that are vital to the generation of the action potential. These channels open or close depending on the state of the membrane electric potential, to allow selective movement of Na^+ or K^+ and generate a traveling action potential, as follows.

Fig. 5-5. Generation of an an axon action potential.

In order to fire a neuron (i.e. create a traveling action potential) the membrane potential must be partially neutralized by some stimulus (whether mechanical, chemical or electrical) to a certain threshold level that is closer to zero than the resting potential. The exact degree of change in potential that is necessary to fire the cell may vary with the type of cell, but it commonly requires a change of about 15–35 millivolts (Fig. 5-3). For example, if the normal potential difference is −60 millivolts, the potential difference may have to be neutralized to −40 millivolts, at which point the local voltage-dependent Na^+ gate suddenly opens and Na^+ rushes into the cell (**depolarization**). This inrush occurs so fast that before the cell has a chance to recover, the inside of the cell may become neutral or even posi-

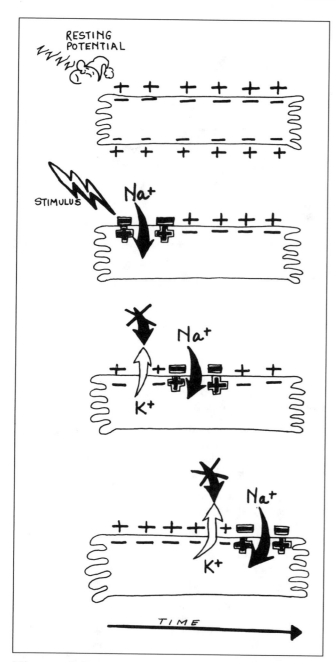

Figure 5-5

gers not only the shutting off of the voltage-dependent sodium gate, but also the opening of a voltage-dependent potassium gate. K^+ thus rushes out quickly to help restore the original membrane potential (**repolarization**). The axon thereby recovers along its length as the action potential travels. The axon cannot fire again until the membrane potential is restored, thus demonstrating a **refractory period**.

In addition to the above-mentioned Na^+ and K^+ gates, there is yet another very important gate, that for calcium (Ca^{++}). Ca^{++} concentration normally is much higher extracellularly than intracellularly due to a calcium pump that pumps calcium out of the cell. Voltage-dependent opening of sodium channels may be accompanied by voltage-dependent opening of calcium channels, which causes further depolarization of the cell membrane. The difference between the sodium and the calcium effect is that calcium channels operate more slowly than do sodium channels. Thus, in cells where the calcium channel mechanism is especially prominent, there is a plateau in the action potential (Fig. 5-3) and recovery of the membrane potential is delayed.

Calcium channels, with their associated plateau effects, are especially prominent in cardiac and smooth muscle cells, where it is desirable to have a relatively prolonged, complete contraction. In contrast, rapid recovery of the membrane potential is desirable for generation of an axon action potential, to ensure that numerous axon potentials can follow rapidly in sequence to relay a coded message; thus, the calcium channels are much less prominent in axons. A plateau is desirable in the spread of impulses in the cardiac Purkinje fibers, because a plateau creates a refractory period during Purkinje fiber discharge that protects the heart against excessively rapid arrhythmias.

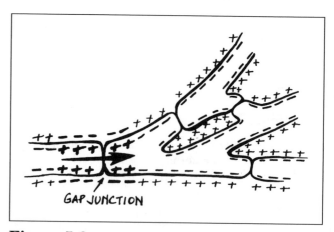

Figure 5-6

tive in relation to the outside. The depolarization spreads laterally to bordering areas of the axon, opening up the neighboring voltage-dependent sodium gates, so that the electrical impulse spreads down the axon (in both directions, if the original stimulus was to the axon itself rather than to the dendrites or cell body).

As quickly as the impulse spreads, the axon recovers, because the neutralized electric potential quickly trig-

Fig. 5-6. Impulse spread in myocardial cells. The depolarization is facilitated by gap junctions between the branched cardiac muscle cells, which bind the cells of the heart into one functional syncytium.

In Fig. 5-3, compare the cell membrane electrical discharge (action potential) in neuron, cardiac conduction system and cardiac muscle:

In Fig. 5-3A, note the rapid ascent (depolarization) and rapid descent (repolarization) of the action potential generated by a **nerve fiber** when it is **stimulated**. This ensures that many impulses can pass in a short time, a requirement for proper neurologic function.

In Fig. 5-3B, note that the action potential generated by the **SA node** is self-generating. No stimulus is necessary, because there is a spontaneous depolarization, as seen in the slow upsweep of the early part of the impulse. In chemical terms, the slow upsweep is the result of a leakiness of the cell membrane to sodium, which seeps into the cell, resulting in the spontaneous action potential. Cells in the AV node (Fig. 5-3D) have similar qualities but are not quite as leaky as SA node cells.

In Fig. 5-3C, note the action potential in an atrial muscle cell, particularly the plateau, which represents the influence of the slow calcium channels and a prolongation of the time of depolarization. This helps to protect against a too rapid heart rate. That is, it allows enough time for the atrial muscle to contract completely and empty the atria. Action potentials in ventricular muscle cells (Fig. 5-3F) have an even more prolonged plateau. The influence of calcium is especially important in muscle cells, since calcium ions activate the interaction between actin and myosin that is necessary for muscular contraction.

In Fig. 5-3E, note the plateau in the action potential generated in the **Purkinje fibers**. It reflects the slow calcium channels and a refractory period, which helps protect against an excessively rapid heart rate and allows time for a full ventricular contraction. Thus, the slow calcium channels are important in regulating both the rate and strength of muscular contraction.

The action potential of **skeletal muscle** has a relatively sharp rise and fall, as does an axon action potential. Thus rapid, successive discharges of a skeletal muscle fiber can result in **tetany**, the cumulation of multiple sustained contractions with no significant relaxation.

The action potential of a smooth muscle cell can resemble that of a skeletal muscle or have a prolonged plateau (e.g. uterine muscle). In the former case, successive rapid depolarizations can, like the skeletal muscle, result in sustained contractions. In the latter, a single depolarization can result in a prolonged contraction.

Smooth muscle cells in blood vessels contract more slowly than cardiac muscle, have a more prolonged action potential and plateau, and are more dependent upon calcium ion influx than are cardiac cells.

Sympathetic stimulation increases both heart rate and myocardial contractility, thereby increasing cardiac output. Parasympathetic stimulation decreases both heart rate and myocardial contractility, but the effect on contractility is much less than that of the sympathetic system, because parasympathetic innervation of the ventricles is minimal, whereas sympathetic fibers innervate all areas of the heart.

Norepinephrine released by sympathetic fibers interacts with beta-1 receptors on cardiac muscle cells, leading to **increased cardiac contractility** by promoting increased calcium influx with each actional potential. Heart rate also increases through **increasing the firing rate of the SA node**, probably by interacting with the permeabilities of Na^+, K^+, and Ca^{++}. Action potential **conduction velocity** also increases.

Parasympathetic fibers, which release acetylcholine, are more selective in their innervation. They decrease cardiac pumping by innervating the SA and AV nodes and the atria. This innervation decreases heart rate (SA node influence), decreases action potential conduction velocity (through the AV node) and decreases the contractility of the atrial muscle (but not ventricular muscle). Acetylcholine increases membrane permeability of the SA node to K^+, thereby hyperpolarizing the cell membranes and rendering them less susceptible to depolarization.

It is important to note that the heart can pump quite well without the pumping action of the atria, as the "suction" generated by ventricular diastole is the main driving force for ventricular filling. Hence, patients with chronic atrial fibrillation can often function quite well. The atrial contraction function becomes more important with vigorous exercise, during which the extra kick to ventricular filling may be particularly helpful.

Cardiac drugs may influence heart rate, rhythm or contractility. Their effects largely are based on several mechanisms:

1) **Interference with the sodium-potassium pump.** For example, digitalis interferes with the sodium-potassium pump, resulting in delayed conduction through the AV node (prolongs the AV node refractory period). This interference may be helpful in slowing dangerous tachycardias like atrial flutter and fibrilla-

tion. Interference with the Na^+/K^+ pump increases intracellular sodium, because sodium is not pumped out of the cell so well. The increased intracellular sodium then exchanges more readily with extracellular Ca^{++}, thereby increasing intracellular Ca^{++}. This increases myocardial contractility, which may be helpful in treating heart failure.

2) **Calcium channel blockers** delay the influx of calcium into the cell. They therefore decrease myocardial contractility and may be useful in decreasing oxygen consumption in angina. The calcium channel blockers, by interfering with smooth muscle contractility, are also useful as vasodilators in treating hypertension and in increasing coronary blood flow. Since the mechanism of SA and AV node pacing depends in part on calcium influx, certain calcium channel blockers (e.g. verapamil and diltiazem) may slow the heart rate if they also delay the recovery of the calcium channel from the depolarization.

3) **Interference with the transmission of autonomic impulses.** In order to understand this, one must first consider the positioning and functions of alpha and beta receptors in the sympathetic nervous system:

Review Fig. 2-5. Note that stimulation of alpha-1, beta-1, and beta-2 receptors will **increase** the sympathetic nerve effects, since sympathetic nerves stimulate these receptors. However, since presynaptic alpha-2 receptors **inhibit** the release of norepinephrine from the presynaptic neuron, stimulating them will **decrease** sympathetic nerve effects. If you wish to inhibit the sympathetic nervous system, you may use alpha-1, beta-1, or beta-2 inhibitors (**antagonists**), or alpha-2 stimulators (**agonists**).

Common uses of autonomic-acting drugs include the following:

1) Alpha-2 **agonists** (e.g. alphamethyldopa, clonidine, guanabenz, guanfacine) may be useful adjuncts in treating hypertension. These drugs decrease peripheral vascular resistance and reduce heart rate and contractility.

2) Alpha-1 **antagonists** (e.g. prazosin, terazosin) reduce blood pressure by decreasing peripheral vascular resistance. Alpha antagonists that nonselectively antagonize both alpha-1 and alpha-2 receptors (e.g. phentolamine, phenoxybenzamine) may also decrease blood pressure by vasodilation. However, such drugs incur the risk of a reflex tachycardia (in response to the decreased blood pressure) by inhibiting alpha-2 receptors in the central nervous system.

3) Reserpine, guanethidine and guanedrel are sympathetic antagonists that enter the postganglionic neuron nerve terminals and block the release of norepinephrine. They may be used to treat hyperten-

sion, but side effects, such as postural hypotension, render them much less desirable than other drugs.

4) Beta blockers not only influence blood pressure but are valuable in treating a variety of cardiac problems, including arrhythmias and cardiac ischemia, since beta receptors influence electrical conduction and muscle contraction within the heart.

Beta-1 blockers decrease heart rate, decrease cardiac contractility and decrease conduction time through the AV node because of the corresponding locations of beta-1 receptors in the heart. These drugs are therefore useful in treating hypertension, through decreased cardiac output (by decreasing heart rate and stroke volume). As beta-1 receptors on kidney granular cells (of the juxtaglomerular apparatus) normally cause renin release when stimulated, beta-1 blockers also reduce blood pressure through inhibition of renin release.

Beta-blockers, by reducing heart rate, cardiac contractility, and afterload (the tension in the ventricular muscle fibers during systolic contraction) also reduce cardiac oxygen demand and can be useful in treating angina. Their use is a two-edged sword, however, since beta blockers can cause heart failure by reducing cardiac output in patients who already have significantly impaired left ventricular function. They can also cause conduction block through slowing of conduction through the AV node.

Beta blockers are useful in treating cardiac arrhythmias as they can reduce a hyperactive automaticity of the SA node as well as ectopic foci of cardiac stimulation. By slowing conduction through the AV node, beta blockers can reduce tachycardias that originate before the AV node, including atrial fibrillation and atrial flutter. They may also help to treat ventricular arrhythmias, such as premature ventricular contractions. The beneficial cardiac effects of beta blockers result in part from the effect of beta blockers on nodal and myocardial beta receptors, but are also due to the reduction on myocardial oxygen demand by reducing blood pressure.

Drugs that nonselectively antagonize both beta-1 and beta-2 receptors incur the risk of inducing bronchospasm and vasospasm, because beta-2 stimulation is important in maintaining broncho-and vasodilation (See Fig. 2-5). Such nonselective drugs must be avoided where possible in patients with asthma or chronic obstructive pulmonary disease (COPD) because they may induce additional bronchospasm. Vasospasm caused by the beta-2 blockade can sometimes be severe enough to cause gangrene in patients who already have peripheral vascular disease. Hence, in treating cardiac disease, it is often desirable to use a beta-blocker that specifically exhibits beta-1, but not beta-2 antagonism.

The picture is complicated by the fact that some beta antagonists can have partial beta agonist qualities or additional alpha-1 blocking capabilities, as well as other peculiar properties. The particular features of each drug must therefore be measured against the particular patient and the problem that one is trying to resolve.

Drugs may improve angina by a number of mechanisms:

1) **Promotion of vasodilation of the coronary arteries**. Nitroglycerin, for example, may reduce vascular tone through the production of nitric oxide.

2) **Reducing preload.** (Preload will be discussed later, but for present purposes it means the tension that arises in the ventricular muscle fibers from expansion of the ventricules during diastole; excess ventricular dilation increases preload.) Nitroglycerin, for example, in addition to its effect on coronary arteries, improves angina partly by dilating systemic veins, so that blood pools in the veins and does not excessively fill the ventricles.

3) **Reducing afterload.** (Afterload is the tension in the ventricular muscle during systolic contraction; it increases with increasing systemic arterial blood pressure, against which the ventricles must strain.)

Afterload may be decreased by reducing arteriolar resistance and blood pressure.

4) **Reducing cardiac contractility and heart rate,** thereby reducing the oxygen need of the heart. **Sympathetic blockers** include beta-blocking drugs such as propranolol. **Calcium channel blockers** (e.g. verapamil) dilate coronary arteries and limit cardiac muscle contractility through interference with the calcium influx that causes muscle contraction.

The Electrocardiogram (ECG)

The ECG is a record of the electrical discharges that occur within the heart through the various phases of the chain of electrical communication within the heart:

Fig. 5-7. Normal components of the ECG. Moving horizontally, each small square represents .04 sec (when the ECG is run at the proper paper speed of 25mm/sec), and each set of 5 small squares thus represents 0.2 sec, important numbers to remember in quantifying ECG results.

P wave: a record of atrial muscle depolarization. (The firing of the SA node does not give a strong enough sig-

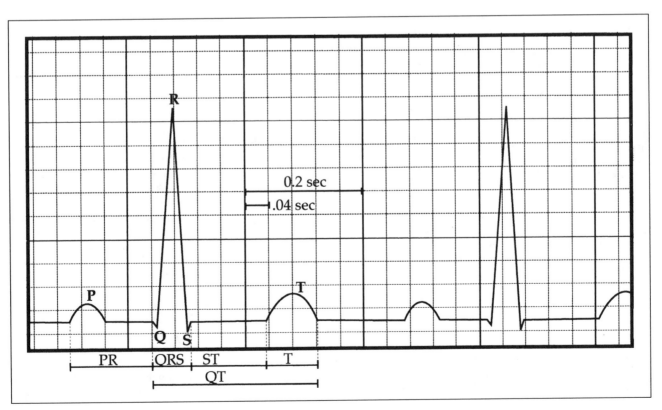

Figure 5-7

nal to be detected in the ECG. Nor is repolarization of the atria detected normally.)

P-R interval: the interval from the **beginning** of the P wave to the **beginning** of the QRS complex. It reflects the time required for conduction of the impulse through the atria, AV node, common bundle, and bundle branches up to the time of ventricular depolarization.

QRS interval: the interval from the **beginning** of the Q wave to the **end** of the S wave. It reflects the depolarization of muscle fibers in the ventricles. The ECG does not record the actual mechanical contraction of muscle fibers, which immediately follows the electrical depolarization of the muscle cells.

S-T segment: the segment between the **end** of the QRS interval and the **beginning** of the T wave. It is the pause between ventricular muscle firing and ventricular muscle repolarization.

T wave: ventricular muscle cell repolarization.

Q-T interval: the interval between the beginning of the QRS and the **end** of the T wave. It represents the duration of ventricular electrical activity.

U wave: not always seen; may be due to repolarization of the bundle branches and Purkinje fibers. It occurs between the T and P waves.

The electrode leads that detect electrical signals from the heart are positioned at various points on the body to "look" at the heart at different angles. The classic 12 electrocardiogram leads are called I, II, III, aVR, aVL, aVF, V1, V2, V3, V4, V5, and V6.

Fig. 5-8. In a very general way, cardiac depolarization spreads from upper right to lower left (in reference to the body as a whole), considering the tilt of the heart. This is important in understanding an overview of the various tracings of the ECG leads.

Fig. 5-9. Positions of the ECG leads. The jagged and straight arrows indicate the axes between the negative and positive electrodes. Cardiac depolarization that spreads in the direction of an arrow, i.e. toward a positive electrode, results in a positive (upward) deflection on the ECG, above the baseline. Impulses traveling away from a positive electrode result in a negative (downward) deflection, below the baseline.

Fig. 5-10. Combined records for leads I, II, III, aVR, aVL, and aVF. The charges on the circle perimeter refer to the charges of the corresponding electrodes. The shaded area indicates the normal directional range of cardiac depolarization, i.e., the normal "axis" of the heart. Since depolarization normally spreads from upper right to lower left, this places the depolarization as

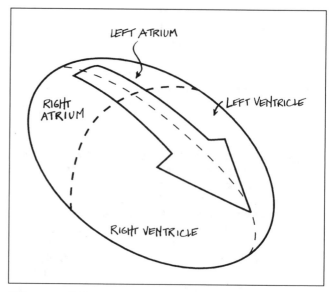

Figure 5-8

spreading, for the most part, toward positive electrodes, except for AVR, and sometimes V1.

Mnemonic for memorizing Fig. 5-10:

aVF: "**F**" in aVF is closest to the **F**oot. Leads aVL and aVR are **L**eft and **R**ight, respectively, in mirror image positions.

"**II**" and "**III**" are heavier than "**I**" so they are near the floor by aVF. "**I**" is higher (on the right).

The net result of the various electrode positions is that the ECG looks at the heart from a variety of positions. Leads I, II, III, aVR, aVL, and aVF look at the heart along the vertical (frontal) plane, whereas leads V1–V6 (Fig. 5-9) look at the heart along the horizontal (transverse) plane.

Fig. 5-11. The normal 12-lead ECG (from ECG INTERPRETATION, by John B. Schwedel, MD, Warner-Chilcott, 1964). Normally, depolarization spreads toward the positive ECG electrodes, except for AVR. Therefore, there tends to be a positive (upward) polarity of the P and QRS waves throughout most ECG leads, except for AVR. In progressing from leads V1 through V6, the overall QRS tends to become progressively more positive, in keeping with the positions of these electrodes in relation to the direction of electrical discharge. The net QRS direction in V1 commonly is down, since the ventricular electrical activity moves left, away from V1. The T wave in V1 can be positive, negative, or biphasic, but is usually positive in V2–V6 in the normal adult. The P wave is consistently positive in lead II in normal adults.

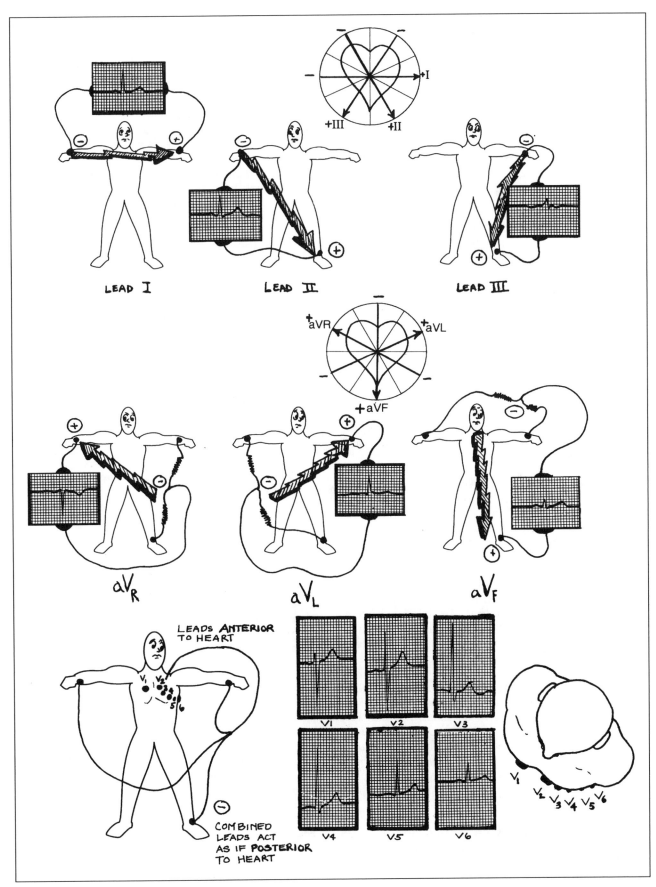

LEAD I   LEAD II   LEAD III

+I

+III   +II

+aVR   +aVL

+aVF

aV$_R$ aV$_L$ aV$_F$

LEADS ANTERIOR TO HEART

COMBINED LEADS ACT AS IF POSTERIOR TO HEART

V1   V2   V3

V4   V5   V6

V$_1$ V$_2$ V$_3$ V$_4$ V$_5$ V$_6$

Figure 5-9

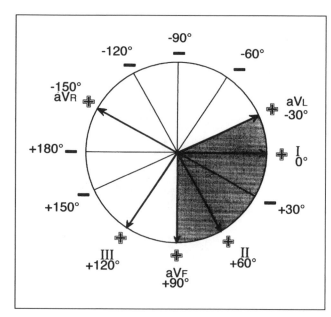

Figure 5-10

Normal variations in the cardiogram arise largely because some hearts lie relatively horizontally and others relatively vertically.

The downward deflection of the Q wave in the QRS complex occurs because septal depolarization proceeds from left to right, arising from connections from the left bundle branch. Ventricular depolarization spreads from the subendocardial surface of the heart to the subepicardial surface.

Fig. 5-12. A simple method for calculating heart rate (modified from ECG INTERPRETATION, by John B. Schwedel, MD, Warner-Chilcott, 1964). The distance markers on the standard ECG encompass 15 large boxes, or 3 seconds. Count the number of QRS complexes between 2 markers and multiply by 20. This gives the number of QRS complexes per 60 seconds and equals the heart rate/minute. More simply (and more accurately), count the number of QRS complexes between 3 markers (6 seconds) and multiply by 10. In Fig. 5-12, there is a "2:1 block" in which only 1 of every 2 P waves gets through the generate a QRS complex. The atrial rate, as measured by the P waves, thus is about 110–120, whereas the ventricular rate, as measured by the QRS complexes, is about 50–60.

The cardiogram can show heart **rate, rhythm, axis** of heart rotation, heart muscle **hypertrophy**, and cardiac muscle ischemia (O_2 deprivation short of tissue death) or **infarction** (tissue death).

Fig. 5-13 (A-Z). Classic disorders of cardiac rate, rhythm, axis, size, ischemia and infarction:

Fig. 5-13 (B-K). Abnormalities in heart rate and rhythm. **Sinus tachycardia** (which may be normal, e.g. in exercise or anxiety) is a rapid heart rate (>100) that originates in the sinoatrial node. In the illustrated case (rate about 150) note that the atrial firing occurs so rapidly that the P waves overlap the T waves. Shown for comparison is a **nodal tachycardia**, in which the AV node is the pacemaker. In this illustrated case, the QRS complexes are not preceded by P waves; instead, the P waves travel retrograde from the AV node and are seen inverted on the T waves. In other cases, the P waves may be before, after, or lost in the QRS complex.

In **first-degree heart block**, the impulses are delayed in getting through the AV node. The P-R interval is >0.20 sec, but the impulses still get through. In **second-degree heart block**, the delay is such that impulses sometimes do not pass through the AV node. There may be P waves with no corresponding QRS complexes. The P:QRS ratio may be 2:1, 3:1, 4:1 or greater. A 2:1 block is illustrated. In **complete heart block**, P waves do not get through the AV nodes; QRS complexes originate from an AV node pacemaker (or ventricles), out of synchrony with the P waves.

Premature ventricular contractions (PVCs) are seen in the ECG as wide, tall, bizarre QRS complexes that arise from ectopic ventricular foci.

Atrial flutter is a rapid, regular succession of discharges from an ectopic atrial focus, fast enough (240–360 waves/min) that the AV node cannot handle all of them. The ECG has a "saw-toothed" pattern.

Atrial fibrillation consists of weak, irregular discharges from a number of atrial foci. There is no discernible P wave, and QRS intervals are irregularly spaced, due to inconsistent transmission of atrial impulses through the AV node.

Ventricular tachycardia consists of a series of rapid, bizarre QRS complexes that originate in the ventricles and become the pacemaker of the heart.

Ventricular fibrillation is a life-threatening, terminal arrhythmia consisting of totally disorganized ventricular discharges from multiple ventricular foci. It results in weak, ineffective contractions of the ventricular muscle.

Fig. 5-13 (L-M). Axis deviations. The normal axis of depolarization lies between −30° and +90°. Thus, if the axis is normal, then ECG leads I and II should show net upward deflections. If either leads I or II show a nega-

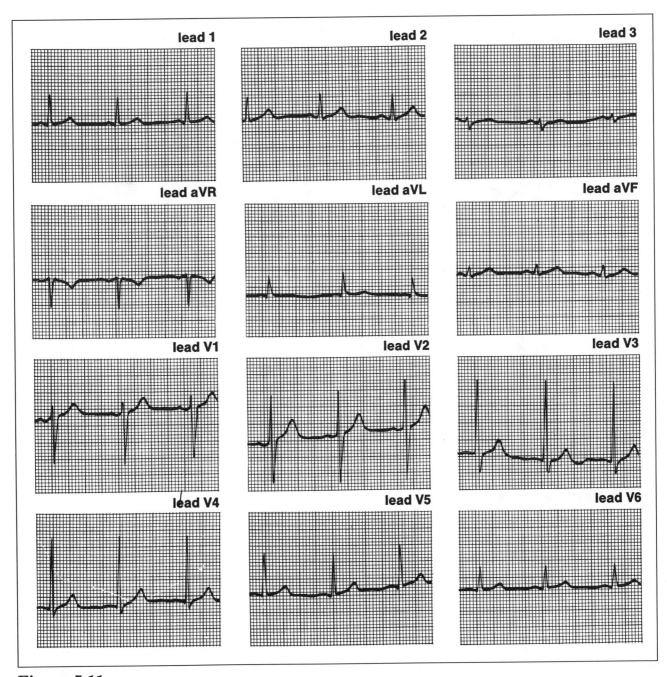

Figure 5-11

tive deflection, then there is an axis deviation. In **left axis deviation**, lead II is negative, whereas lead I is negative in **right axis deviation**. Such axis deviations may result from ventricular hypertrophy (e.g. left ventricular hypertrophy may be associated with left axis deviation in the 0° to −30° range, whereas right ventricular hypertrophy may be associated with right axis deviation) or from infarctions or blocks in the conduc-

tion system that cause rerouting of the spread of electrical activity.

Fig. 5-13 (N-Q). Cardiac hypertrophy. In **left atrial hypertrophy**, or dilatation, the P wave may be "M-shaped" and broad in lead II, and biphasic with a significant negative component in V1, reflecting the delayed spread of impulses to an enlarged left atrium.

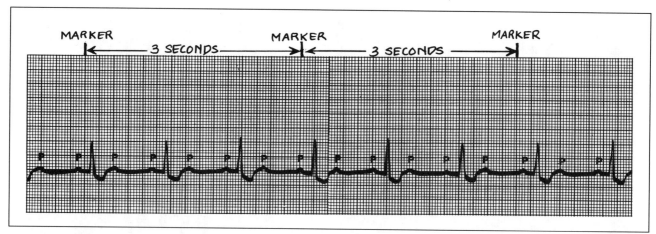

Figure 5-12

In **right atrial hypertrophy** or dilatation the amplitude of the P wave increases.

Ventricular hypertrophy is manifested as an increased amplitude of the QRS complex. Normally, the electrical activity of the left ventricle is more prominent than that of the right. Thus, in the normal ECG, the net QRS deflection in V1 is down, reflecting the spread of ventricular electrical activity **away** from V1 (which lies near the right ventricle), whereas the net deflection in V6 is up, reflecting the spread of ventricular activity **toward** V6 (which lies near the left ventricle). In left ventricular hypertrophy, these deflections are increased still further in amplitude. In **right ventricular hypertrophy**, there is a reversal of this; the net deflection is up in V1, reflecting the spread of electrical activity mainly toward the right ventricle, whereas the net deflection is decreased in V6, reflecting the spread of electrical activity largely away from the left ventricle.

Fig. 5-13 (R-T). Ischemia (tissue anoxia short of death) and infarction (tissue death). In general, elevation of the ST segment, followed by T wave inversion, are ischemic changes that may proceed to full infarction. The development of deep Q waves signifies infarction. Whereas ST elevation and T wave inversion may ultimately disappear, Q waves persist as an indicator of a previous myocardial infarction.

The diagnoses of ischemia and infarction and their precise location depend on the leads that show the abnormalities. Although there are physiologic explanations as to why there are particular patterns that involve particular leads in the various kinds of infarction, one reaches a point where it is simply easier to remember the patterns than to go through the logic of figuring them out from the mechanisms. A few common

patterns are as follows: Wider than normal Q waves in leads II, III, and aVF suggest **inferior wall** infarction (the inferior wall is the diaphragmatic surface of the heart). Q waves in V1–V2 commonly occur in **anteroseptal** infarcts. Q waves in V5–V6, I and aVL commonly occur in **anterolateral** infarction.

Fig. 5-13 (U-V). Bundle branch blocks. Blocks in electrical transmission along the right or left bundles cause rerouting of discharges to the ventricles. Among other things, this causes a peculiar notched appearance in the QRS, more prominent in V5–V6 in **left bundle branch block**, and more prominent in V1–V2 in right **bundle branch block**, as illustrated in the figure.

Fig. 5-13 (W-Z). Metabolic abnormalities seen on the ECG. Note the tall, peaked T waves in **hyperkalemia**; U wave and flat T wave in **hypokalemia**; short Q-T interval in **hypercalcemia**, and prolonged Q-T interval in **hypocalcemia**.

Heart Sounds

Fig. 5-14. The major events on the left side of the heart during a cardiac cycle. Details for the right side of the heart are qualitatively similar. **Mnemonic:** Imagine a "Y" between S1 and S2 to give S1YS2, indicating that systole (SYS) occurs between the first (S1) and second (S2) heart sounds. The figure will help us to understand the reason behind the murmurs heard in certain cardiac conditions. Note that heart sounds normally result from valve closure. Valve opening is not normally heard. Thus, the first heart sound reflects closure of the atrioventricular (tricuspid and mitral) valves during systole. The second heart sound reflects closure of the semilunar (pulmonary and aortic) valves during diastole.

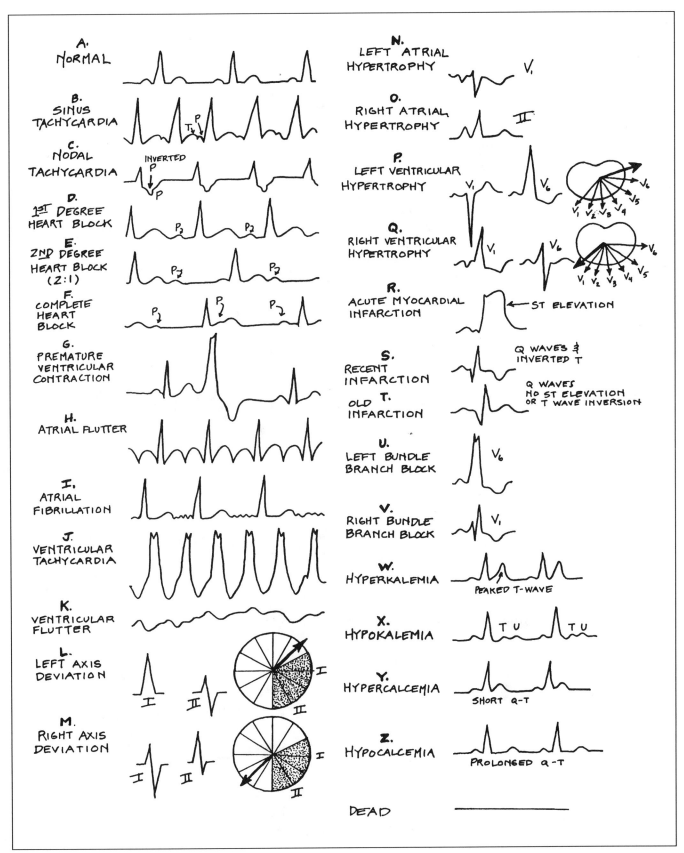

Figure 5-13

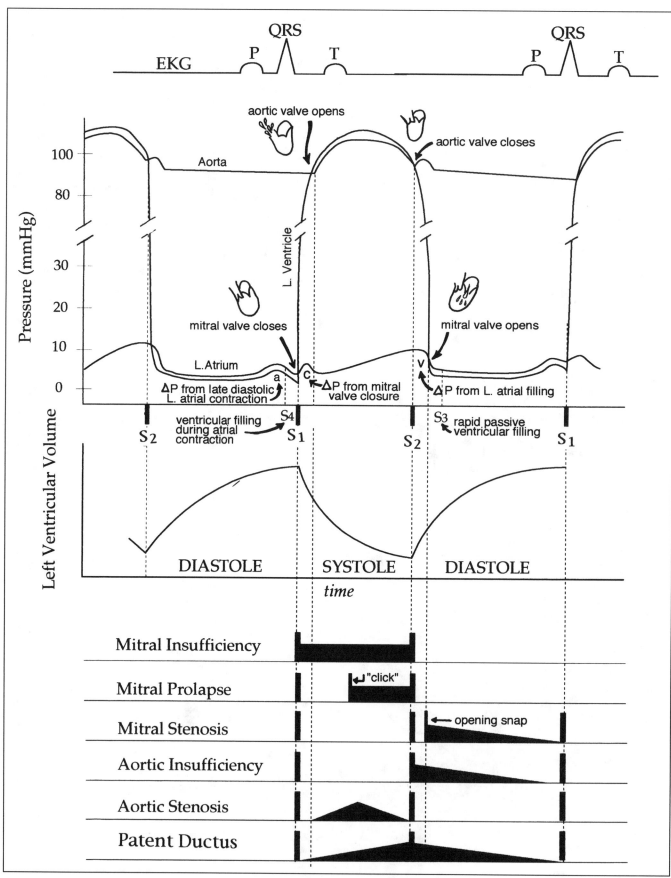

Figure 5-14

The S3 and S4 heart sounds normally are not heard through the stethescope, although the S3 may heard in normal children and young adults. S3 represents rapid **passive** ventricular filling, occurring when the ventricles begin to expand during diastole. S3 is heard pathologically in older adults with ventricular failure as a "ventricular gallop," sounding like "Ken-**tuc**-ky," the three syllables representing S1,S2 and S3 respectively. The ventricles generally are overfilling in an S3 murmur.

S4 represents rapid **active** ventricular filling, which occurs when the atria contract and empty in the latter part of ventricular diastole. An S4 may be heard in various cardiac diseases as an "atrial gallop," sounding like "Ten-nes-**see**," reflecting S4, S1, and S2 in sequence. The ventricles generally are stiff and resistant to dilation (e.g. ventricular hypertrophy) in an S4 murmur.

Note that because of the high pressure in the aorta, the aortic valve opens after the mitral valve closes, and closes before the mitral valve opens. Thus the aortic valve is open for a shorter time than is the mitral valve.

Note in Fig. 5-14 that there are atrial "a," "c," and "v" pressure waves. The "a" wave relects a rise in atrial pressure during late diastolic atrial contraction. The "c" wave occurs after closure of the A-V valves during systole. The "v" wave arises from atrial filling during systole. The "a" wave is commonly transmitted to the jugular vein, where it can be observed on the patient's neck at the bedside, preceeding the common carotid artery pulse. This can provide useful information about the patient's cardiac status. For instance, there may be a very large "a" wave in pulmonary artery stenosis. Giant irregular "a" wave pulses may occur in third-degree heart block, where atrial contraction may occur at the same time as right ventricular contraction; in that case, the tricuspid valve remains closed during right atrial contraction. A systolic wave in the neck is seen in tricuspid insufficiency at about the same time as cardiac sound S1, due to regurgitation of blood back into the right atrium during systole.

Most of the filling of the ventricles occurs during the first third of diastole, and most of the emptying of the ventricles occurs during the first third of systole. That

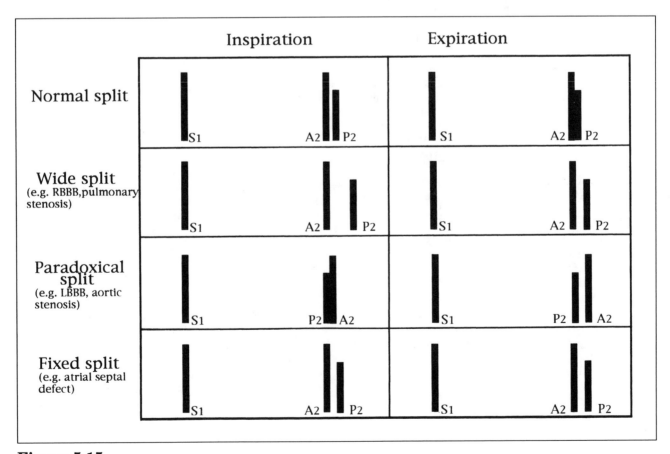

Figure 5-15

is, blood flow in the ventricles is relatively fast during the first third of diastole and systole. Therefore, in aortic valve insufficiency, the backflow insufficiency murmur is loudest during the first part of diastole. (However, the murmur of mitral insufficiency characteristically is plateau-shaped throughout systole). The insufficiency murmurs are relatively high-pitched, due to the high velocity of blood flow.

In mitral and aortic stenosis, there is little murmur immediately after S1 or S2, because S1 and S2 represent **closure** of the mitral and aortic valves respectively, whereas these murmurs begin with the **opening** of the mitral valve (mitral stenosis) and aortic valve (aortic stenosis), events which slightly follow the opposite valve closures. That is, aortic valve opening follows the S1 of mitral valve closure, and mitral valve opening follows the S2 of aortic valve closure (review Fig. 5-14).

Fig. 5-14, as mentioned, depicts events on the **left** side of the heart, including information relating to the left atrium, mitral valve, left ventricle, aortic valve and aorta. The graph for the right side of the heart (i.e. information relating to the right atrium, tricuspid valve, right ventricle, pulmonary valve, and pulmonary artery) is not shown but is qualitatively similar. Events on the right side of the heart occur roughly at the same time as corresponding events on the left side. Quantitatively, though, there are important differences. For one, the pressure in the pulmonary artery (mean about 16mm Hg) is markedly less than that in the aorta (mean about 100mm Hg). Moreover, whereas the tricuspid and mitral valves close at essentially the same time, the aortic and pulmonary valves do not quite do so, leading (in inspiration) to splitting of the second heart sound.

Fig. 5-15. Splitting of the S2 heart sounds. The aortic valve normally closes slightly before the pulmonary valve (as one might expect, given the large back pressure of the aorta). This difference in closure times is most pronounced during inspiration, where the negative pressure during inspiration increases the inflow to the right side of the heart and decreases inflow from the lungs to the left atrium and ventricle). The resultant increased volume within the right ventricle and decreased volume of the left ventricle result in a more prolonged right ventricular contraction and, hence, a delay in the closure of the pulmonary valve during inspiration. During expiration, the closure sounds during S2 should coincide (Fig. 5-15).

Knowledge of the splitting sequence is important clinically. In **right bundle branch block**, the right ventricle is slow in contracting and there is a delay in pulmonary valve closure, leading to a wide split in the S2 sound. In **left bundle branch block**, the left ventricle is slow in contracting and there is a **paradoxical split** of S2, in which the aortic valve closes **after** the pulmonary valve during both expiration and inspiration. In that case, the split paradoxically increases in expiration and **decreases** or disappears during inspiration.

Delay of closure of the pulmonary valve, with consequent sound splitting effects, may also be observed in pulmonary stenosis (blood then takes extra time to get through the pulmonary valve), whereas closure of the aortic valve may be delayed in aortic stenosis. The S2 sound itself may increase in loudness in forced closure of the pulmonary valve in pulmonary hypertension, or aortic valve in aortic hypertension.

Preload and Afterload

A muscle undergoes an **isometric** ("same-length") contraction when it maintains a fixed length during the course of contraction. An example is the simultaneous contraction of biceps and triceps muscle so that there is no net movement at the elbow, even though the tension in each muscle increases. In an **isotonic** ("same strength") contraction, the muscle shortens as it tightens, maintaining the same tension during the course of movement. An example is the contraction of the biceps muscle alone, which causes the bending of the elbow. Part of cardiac contraction is isometric, and part is isotonic. In diastole, the increased volume of the ventricles expands the cardiac wall. At the outset of systole, there is an initial isometric contraction against this increased volume. This is followed by opening of the semilunar valves and an isotonic contraction, which forces the blood out of the ventricles.

Imagine a circle of people, all holding hands. Suddenly, a giant balloon appears in the center of the circle and begins expanding, to such a degree that it pushes against all the people, forcing them outward. Since the people are holding hands, the pressure from the balloon, acting at right angles to the people, causes a passive increase in tension in the people's arms, the force of the tension being at right angles to the centrifugal pressure of the balloon.

The increased tension in the people's arms corresponds to the **preload**. Preload is the increase in tension in ventricular cardiac muscle fibers when the ventricle expands in diastole. This passive increase in tension is the result of the increasing volume of the ventricles during diastole.

Now imagine that the circle of people try to resist the balloon by contracting their muscles, forcing the balloon inward, to the point where it explodes, enabling the circle to decrease in diameter.

The increased tension in the people's arms during this active contraction corresponds to the **afterload**. Afterload is the increase in tension in the ventricular cardiac muscle fibers when they actively contract against the expanded ventricular volume to expel the blood through the aortic valve.

Increasing the preload or the afterload increases the energy demands on the heart. This may be more clearly understood through the **Laplace equation** which states that

$$T = Pr$$

where, in the case of the heart, T = the tension of the cardiac muscle, P = intraventricular pressure, and r = radius of the ventricle. Imagine that toward the end of ventricular diastole, the intraventricular pressure is P, the muscle tension is T and the ventricular radius is r. Imagine now, for the sake of argument, that the aortic pressure is $25P$. In order then for the ventricle to expel the blood into the aorta, it has to generate a pressure of $25P$. Then, since $25T = 25Pr$, the tension in the ventricular musculature must increase 25-fold to $25T$ to expel the blood. Thus, you can see that increasing the systemic blood pressure increases the afterload on the heart.

Imagine now that the patient has an abnormally increased systemic blood volume, and the ventricular radius is $2r$ at the end of diastole, but the aortic pressure is still $25P$. The equation now is $50T = 25P(2r)$. In other words, in order for the ventricle to expel the blood against the aortic pressure of $25P$, it has to generate a tension of $50T$, a significant increase. Thus, increasing the radius of the ventricle (commonly through increasing systemic blood volume) will increase not only the preload, but also the afterload and the energy demand on the heart.

Most myocardial oxygen consumption occurs during the isometric phase of cardiac contraction. This would be expected since the ventricular radius decreases as contraction proceeds; the smaller radius, according to the Laplace equation, decreases the tension that the heart muscle has to generate to expel the blood against the aortic pressure.

In summary, in **T** = Pr, an increase in **P** increases the afterload, and an increase in **r** increases the preload. An increase in either will increase T, thereby increasing oxygen demand.

Increased blood pressure **increases** afterload and **decreases** cardiac stroke volume because the ventricle encounters resistance in contracting against an increased systemic blood pressure. **Increased** blood volume **increases** preload and **increases** cardiac stroke volume, as there is increased ventricular filling. One might consider such increased stroke volume as a good thing, but it can contribute to hypertension, in addition to increasing the oxygen demands on the heart.

Diuretics, which decrease blood volume, may be useful in congestive heart failure by decreasing preload. Drugs that reduce systemic blood pressure reduce afterload.

In general, it is more energy efficient for a heart to beat at a relatively low rate with higher stroke volume than for the heart to exhibit the same cardiac output, but with high rate and low stroke volume. Therefore, a drug such as digitalis, which increases stroke volume and decreases heart rate, promotes more efficient cardiac oxygen utilization.

A drug that increases the strength of the heart's contraction is said to have a **positive inotropic** effect. Drugs that increase heart rate have a positive **chronotropic** effect. Drugs that increase conduction velocity have a positive **dromotropic** effect.

Cardiac output may be measured through application of the Fick principle. See the preceeding discussion of the Fick principle used in this regard, in the Blood Pressure chapter). Cardiac output can also be assessed by injecting dye into the venous circulation and measuring its dilutional change per unit time as it enters the arterial circulation.

Normal cardiac output varies with an individual's weight. The **cardiac index**, the cardiac output per square meter of body surface area, is considered a better measure of normal cardiac output than is body weight.

The **ejection fraction** = (stroke volume)/(end-diastolic volume). It is a reflection of cardiac function. In failing hearts, the end-diastolic volume may increase as the stroke volume decreases. The ejection fraction is thus low, indicating poor cardiac pumping action. Information about the ejection fraction can be obtained through a variety of imaging techniques:

In **cardiac angiography**, contrast material is injected through a catheter in the right or left ventricle and one can visualize a moving picture of cardiac function on X-ray. In **echocardiography**, reflected sound wave recordings provide a moving picture of cardiac function. In **radionucleotide ventriculography**, a radioactive substance that is injected intravenously can be detected over the ventricles, providing information about cardiac chamber size and contractility.

CHAPTER 6. THE RESPIRATORY SYSTEM

Pulmonary respiration entails the acquisition of oxygen and release of excess CO_2. The process also adjusts the pH of the blood, since CO_2 and water form a weak acid.

What Muscles Control Respiration?

The main muscle of **inspiration** is the diaphragm. Contraction and downward motion of the diaphragm causes a negative pressure in the chest, which draws in air. Other than the diaphragm, there are accessory muscles of inspiration (pectoralis major and minor, serratus anterior, sternocleidomastoid, scalene muscles, levatores costarum, serratus posterior superior). They may be vital to survival in certain chronic pulmonary diseases.

Expiration is largely passive. Simply by relaxing, the chest springs back into shape, and expiration can occur without any muscle action. (One can, however, voluntarily exhale forcefully, using the external and internal intercostal muscles, the transversus thoracis and innermost intercostal muscles, external oblique, internal oblique and transversus abdominis muscles.)

How Does Hemoglobin Affect Gas Exchange?

Oxygen is not very soluble in plasma. Most oxygen (about 97% of it) is transported via hemoglobin, which has special oxygen-binding capabilities. Consider what special oxygen-binding qualities you would like hemoglobin to have to function efficiently. You would want it to bind to significant quantities of oxygen at the alveolar level, even when oxygen concentration in the alveoli is relatively low. You would, on the other hand, also like hemoglobin to release oxygen easily at the tissue level, but in just the right amounts, since too much can cause oxygen toxicity, and too little will not provide enough for the respiratory needs of the tissue. You would like hemoglobin to release large quantities of oxygen when the tissues really need it. But how can hemoglobin bind well to oxygen in the alveoli, yet release it easily at the peripheral tissue level?

Indeed, hemoglobin does these things, as illustrated by the nonlinearity of the hemoglobin-oxygen dissociation curve.

Fig. 6-1. Oxygen dissociation curve for hemoglobin. Note that hemoglobin maintains near saturation (above 90% saturated) even when alveolar oxygen decreases from the normal 104mm Hg to 60mm Hg. However, when hemoglobin encounters the low tissue pO_2 of the body tissues (normally about 40 mm Hg in interstitial

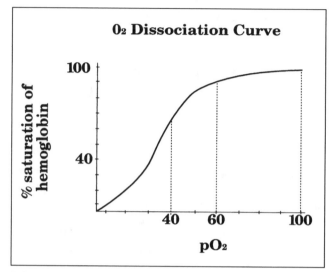

Figure 6-1

fluid), it readily gives up the oxygen, doing so even more vigorously when the pO_2 falls to 20, as might occur during marked exercise. Thus hemoglobin loads up well on oxygen even when faced with marked fluctuations in alveolar pO_2, and it maintains the body tissue requirements for O_2 in the face of marked fluctuations in tissue pO_2 levels.

For added protection, hemoglobin releases more oxygen when the pCO_2 is elevated or the pH is low (conditions that may coincide with anoxia), or when the temperature is elevated (where oxygen needs may be increased).

Considering the oxygen dissociation curve, however, note that if alveolar pO_2 levels fall really low, particularly below 40 (e.g. at an altitude of 20,000 feet, or in other conditions where adequate amounts of oxygen do not reach the alveoli) hemoglobin will falter in trapping oxygen and the patient will go downhill.

Hemoglobin does not transport most of the carbon dioxide. Rather, CO_2 combines with water in the red blood cell (RBC) to form H_2CO_3 (the enzyme carbonic anhydrase in the RBC catalyzes this reaction). The H^+ from the H_2CO_3 combines with the hemoglobin; HCO_3^- leaves the cell and floats around in the blood until the blood reaches the lungs. Then the hemoglobin releases the H^+, which combines with bicarbonate ion to reform CO_2, which is then expelled by the lungs. Some CO_2 does, however, combine directly with hemoglobin (about

25%) to form **carbaminohemoglobin**, which releases its CO_2 in the lungs. Additionally, a small amount of CO_2 (about 5%) dissolves directly in the plasma.

When CO_2 dissolves in the RBC fluid at the capillary level, the HCO_3^- that leaves the red blood cell exchanges with chloride, to maintain ionic charge neutrality. This process reverses in the lungs. Therefore, the chloride content of venous RBCs is greater than that of arterial RBCs (the **chloride shift**).

Apart from hemoglobin, the body's cells are pretty smart in controlling the amount of O_2 that they use. They don't just gobble up all the available oxygen. The rate-limiting step in the cell's utilization of oxygen is not the pO_2, but the level of ADP. The cell needs oxygen to form its energy currency, ATP, from ADP during oxidative phosphorylation. If the level of ADP is low (i.e., the level of ATP is high), the cell doesn't need as much O_2, and less O_2 reacts during oxidative phosphorylation. If the level of ADP is high (i.e., the level of ATP is low), the cell needs to utilize more oxygen to form ATP, and more O_2 reacts during oxidative phosphorylation. Also, increased ATP levels act as a feedback to suppress the cell's utilization of oxygen in the Krebs cycle.

Fig. 6-2. Use of oxygen in the conversion of ADP to ATP in the mitochondria (O_2 is at the end of the chain).

What Neural Factors Control Respiration?

The phrenic nerve (C3,4,5) innervates the diaphragm and receives voluntary and involuntary respiratory messages from the central nervous system. Respiratory centers in the brain stem medulla and pons help control the involuntary aspects of respiration. The brain stem receives feedback in a number of ways:

1) **Carbon dioxide and H+**. Increased blood CO_2 or H^+ levels stimulate the brain stem respiratory centers to increase respiration to blow off CO_2 and decrease blood acidity. The increased CO_2 and decreased pH also stimulate increased firing of the aortic and carotid bodies, which relay neural messages to the brain stem via cranial nerves 9 and 10, to increase respiration. H^+ and CO_2 levels, though, have minimal effects on the carotid and aortic bodies in comparison with their direct effects on the brain stem.

2) **Oxygen**. Decreased blood pO_2 levels increase firing of the carotid and aortic bodies, which relay the information about the state of blood oxygenation to the brain stem.

3) In exercise, it is believed that the **motor cortex** sends direct innervation to stimulate the brain stem respiratory centers at the same time that the brain sends impulses to the skeletal muscles to engage in exercise. In addition, proprioceptive information from the contracting skeletal muscles, and possibly nerve impulses generated locally from skeletal hypoxia, return to the brain stem to stimulate the respiratory center.

4) The **Hering-Breuer** inflation reflex. Stretch receptors in the bronchiolar and bronchial tree send inhibitory impulses to the brain stem that limit excessive inspiration (and simultaneously increase the rate of inspiration).

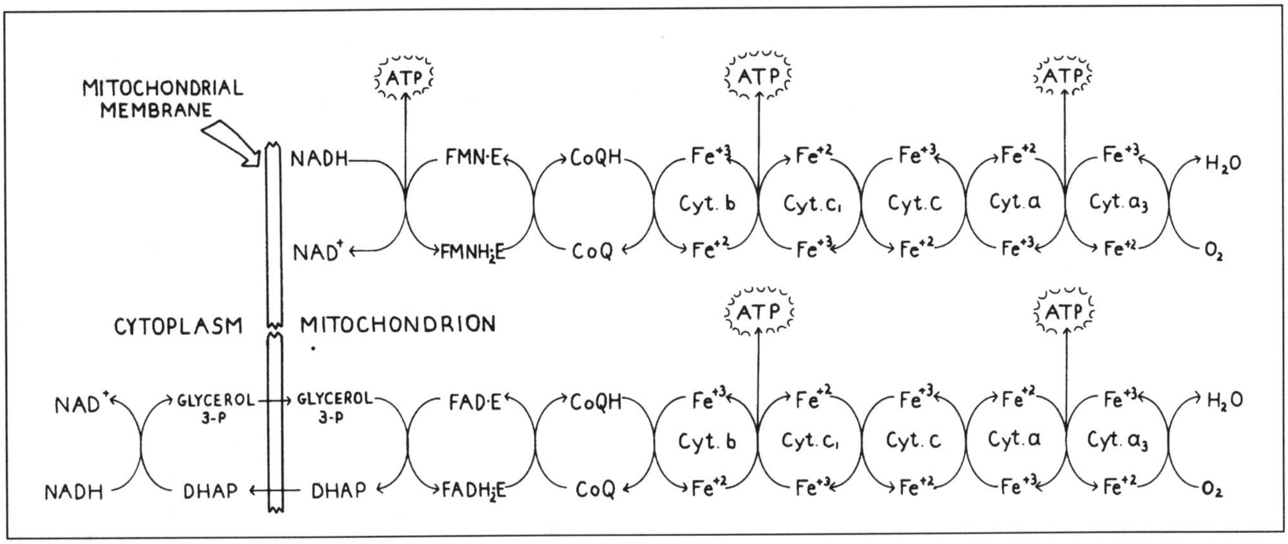

Figure 6-2

CHAPTER 6. THE RESPIRATORY SYSTEM

A moderate increase of pCO_2 stimulates respiration much more than does a moderate decrease in pO_2. So why do we need the O_2 response mechanism? Wouldn't it suffice to just have the pCO_2 control mechanism? Answer: It is true that **moderate** increases in pCO_2 result in increased respiratory rate, without requiring much assistance from the stimulus of decreased O_2. However, in **severe** pulmonary disease, in which there is poor exchange in both O_2 and CO_2, the CO_2 effect is not enough. The large drop in pO_2 then comes into play, having a marked effect in increasing the rate of respiration when the PO_2 falls to the 30–60 mm Hg range.

Another way that O_2 lack becomes important in stimulating respiration is in adaptation to high altitude. The CO_2 blood levels in these conditions may be low or normal, because hyperventilation drives off the CO_2. If pCO_2 levels were the only stimulus to respiration, the respiratory stimulus might stop with the return of pCO_2 levels to normal. However, there is still a need for increased ventilation because of the low supply of oxygen. Similarly, in certain pulmonary diseases, such as pneumonia, CO_2 is easily blown off, but O_2 has difficulty getting in (as CO_2 dissolves much better in water than does O_2, and CO_2 is thus better at getting through the waterlogged alveoli). In such cases, CO_2 levels may be normal or low, and the stimulus to increased respiration may come largely from low blood pO_2.

Then why do we need the CO_2 control mechanism? Why does it not suffice to just control respiration according to the O_2 level? After all, isn't it really the O_2 that the body needs? Shouldn't O_2 levels alone provide the best feedback control? Answer: the CO_2 control mechanism is actually needed more for the control of blood pH than for control of respiration. Subtle changes in the pCO_2 can significantly affect pH, so the body needs the fine CO_2 control mechanism to control CO_2 levels and thus control pH. The O_2 control mechanism is a much cruder mechanism and is inadequate to maintain appropriate CO_2 levels and pH. Consider, for instance, if respiration is failing and alveolar pO_2 falls from 104mm Hg to 60 mm Hg at the same time that body pCO_2 is increasing. If all the body had to rely upon were the O_2 control mechanism, it would scarcely have a clue that anything was happening, since hemoglobin would still be close to O_2 saturation (see Fig. 6-1). The pCO_2 and body pH would remain abnormally acidotic if there were no feedback from pCO_2 levels. Thus both the O_2 and pCO_2 control mechanisms are important.

Breathing high-pressure oxygen (above atmospheric pressure) can markedly increase the saturation of oxygen in the blood, even to toxic levels, not by increased uptake by hemoglobin, but by dissolving more of it in plasma. Breathing air with increased oxygen concen-

tration, but at atmospheric pressure, may slightly increase plasma oxygen, but not by much, since oxygen doesn't dissolve well in plasma, and RBCs are already pretty saturated at normal oxygen concentrations. Simple hyperventilation does not significantly affect plasma (or hemoglobin) oxygenation, since the hemoglobin is already near saturation. **Deep** hyperventilation, however, may help you hold your breath longer, because it expands the lungs and also replaces with fresh air some of the tracheal and bronchial low-O_2 **dead space** (the region in the respiratory tree in which no gas exchange occurs); this puts more reserve air in the lung to use while the breath is held. Deep hyperventilation, however, also blows off CO_2, which may lead to dizziness and in some cases loss of the respiratory reflexes due to the lack of H^+ and CO_2 stimuli to respiration.

If you want to increase tissue oxygenation, you are going to have to increase one of the following: the oxygen concentration in the air being breathed, the hemoglobin concentration, or the blood flow (as by increasing cardiac output). Hyperventilation is not good enough.

Effect Of Altitude On Changes In Respiration

In **diving**, the alveolar pressure rises to meet the increasing atmospheric pressure that results with greater depth. Diving compresses the body tissues, including the air spaces, resulting in more concentrated gases, at higher pressures. The higher pressures cause more nitrogen to be dissolved, which may cause nitrogen toxicity. Oxygen toxicity may also occur, but CO_2 toxicity is not likely because the CO_2 continues to be made in the body in fixed amounts and is expired as needed.

On rising from a dive, it is important that the diver gradually let out air. Otherwise, the lungs will continue to expand against the decreasing outside environmental pressure, thereby causing lung injury. The diver may experience **bends (decompression sickness)** on rising too rapidly through the water. The acutely lower outside atmospheric pressure results in dissolved compressed nitrogen coming out of solution and expanding to form bubbles (like soda fizzing on opening the bottle). The nitrogen bubbles may severely compromise many areas of the body.

Normal air outside the body consists of about 20% oxygen, 79% nitrogen, 0.04% carbon dioxide and <1% water (variable, depending on humidity); it exerts a pressure of 760mm Hg at sea level. The pressure of alveolar air at sea level must also be 760 mm Hg but differs in composition from atmospheric air since it includes water vapor from the body (about 6%), in addition to in-

	ATMOSPHERIC AIR (SEA LEVEL)		ALVEOLAR AIR (SEA LEVEL)	
	%	mm Hg	%	mm Hg
N	78.6	597	74.2	569
O	20	159	74.2	104
CO_2	.04	0.3	3.6	40
H_2O	.50	3.7	6.2	47
TOTAL	100%	760mm Hg	100%	760mm Hg

Figure 6-3

creased CO_2 (6%) and decreased O_2 (15%) from respiratory activity.

Fig. 6-3. Components of alveolar and atmospheric air.

At **high altitudes**, as in low altitudes, the alveolar pressure in normal breathing cannot be more than the atmospheric pressure. Alveolar water vapor pressure remains at about 47mm Hg even at high altitudes, and alveolar pCO_2 does not drop much (about 40 mm Hg to 24 mm Hg) because water and CO_2 are constantly being produced in the body. Thus, the alveolar H_2O and CO_2 pressures in themselves total about 71mm Hg. But at 50,000 feet the total barometric pressure (and hence alveolar pressure) may be as low as 87 mm Hg. Subtracting the contribution of H_2O and CO_2 (71mm Hg), this leaves only 16 mm Hg for other gases. Even if one eliminated N_2 by breathing pure oxygen at that altitude (alveolar pO_2 will then be 16mm Hg), it would not supply enough oxygen to adequately oxygenate the blood. Since part of the alveolar pressure has to be due to water vapor and CO_2, this leaves only a little left for O_2 at high altitudes.

As one climbs to higher elevation, one can at first compensate for decreased atmospheric oxygenation by hyperventilation and later by breathing pure O_2, but above 45,000 feet or so, the atmospheric pressure is so low that even pure O_2 cannot provide enough oxygen saturation to the blood, since the alveolar pO_2 is so low. The body's long range compensation to high altitude may occur initially through hyperventilation, and over weeks to months, through increased tissue vascularity and increased numbers of red blood cells.

Respiratory Problems

Respiratory deficit can occur at any of several levels:

1) A problem with **inspiratory muscles** or **neurogenic control of respiration** (e.g. stroke, brain stem edema from brain injury, drug overdosage, amyotrophic lateral sclerosis, spinal cord injury, polio).

Fig. 6-4. Classic patterns of breathing in brain stem injury. In **Cheyne-Stokes respiration**, there is an overcompensation of deep, rapid breathing, which leads to decreased CO_2 and shutoff of respiration. This, in turn, leads to a buildup again of CO_2 and return of the overcompensated breathing pattern.

2) **Pneumothorax:** air abnormally enters the pleural space. This causes lung collapse and does not allow the necessary negative pressure to develop inside the lung during inspiratory diaphragmatic contraction.

3) Problem of **obstruction** of respiratory passages, such as a foreign body lodged in a bronchus.

4) Problem at **alveolar level:**

a) Too thick a membrane for gas to diffuse through well (e.g. in pulmonary edema)

b) Fluid in alveolar space (e.g. pulmonary edema, pneumonia)

c) Diminished surface area through collapse or replacement of the alveolar space (atelectasis, pulmonary fibrosis, emphysema, invasive tumor). In **emphysema** there is alveolar destruction, decreased alveolar surface area, and decreased gas exchange. Oxygen uptake and CO_2 release are poor. The number of pulmonary capillaries also decreases, resulting in increased pulmonary blood flow resistance, pulmonary hypertension, and right heart failure.

The patient may compensate for poor alveolar ventilation by increasing breathing depth and rate. If the respiratory problem is especially severe, however, the work of breathing in itself may require so much oxygen that the effort fails and the patient may require mechanical ventilation.

One must be cautious in a too rapid lowering of pCO_2 by mechanical ventilation. The resulting alkalosis may cause cerebral vasoconstriction and coma. When the patient ventilates on her own, the decreased pCO_2 (increased pH) normally acts to inhibit the respiratory center and control the pH. Under artificial ventilation, however, the control is not there and should be approached slowly to allow the body's normal buffering

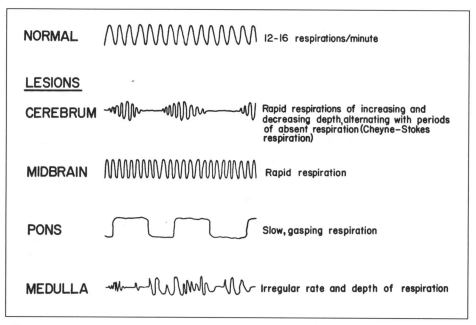

Figure 6-4

mechanisms to come into play and return the pH toward normal.

5) **Poor pulmonary blood flow.** It is relatively uncommon for a low arterial pO_2 to be purely the result of a primary failure of oxygen to diffuse across the alveolar membrane. Rather, a mismatched (air ventilation)/(blood perfusion) ratio, whether low (e.g. due to poor ventilation, pneumonia) or high (due to poor blood perfusion) are the most common causes of arterial hypoxemia.

CO_2 diffuses much better than O_2 between air and the blood because it is far more soluble than O_2. Therefore, patients may develop oxygen diffusion problems, with anoxia, before they develop CO_2 retention.

6) **Inefficient cardiovascular perfusion of the tissues.** This may be a primary pathological problem, as occurs in blood vessel disease or cardiac insufficiency, or a temporary manifestation of marked exercise. When oxygen supply cannot meet the tissue energy needs during marked exercise, the body switches to anaerobic metabolism, rather than the oxygen-dependent Krebs cycle. This is energy inefficient, however, and the individual is also limited by the accumulation of lactate and hydrogen ions in the muscle, with compensatory hyperventilation.

7) **Problem at cell level of gas exchange** (e.g., anemia, carbon monoxide poisoning).

Evaluation Of Pulmonary Function

Arterial blood gas analysis is an important tool in the evaluation of pulmonary function (see Fig. 3-6 and related text for discussion of metabolic versus respiratory acidosis and alkalosis). Proper interpretation of blood gases requires a knowledge of normal lab values for arterial pH, HCO_3^-, pO_2 and pCO_2. Normal arterial pH is about 7.35–7.45. Normal serum $HCO3^-$ is about 24–28meq/L. Normal arterial pO_2 is about 95mm Hg (normal range 80–100mm Hg at sea level) and normal arterial pCO_2 is about 40mm Hg (normal range about 35–45mm Hg).

Fig. 6-5. The pO_2 and pCO_2 levels in the atmosphere and body. The pO_2 averages about 23mm Hg at the peripheral **intracellular level**, but not to worry—the cell needs a pO_2 of only about 2mm Hg for adequate functioning.

The pulmonary capillary pO_2 and pCO_2 equilibrate with alveolar pO_2 and pCO_2 after passing about 1/3 of the way through the pulmonary capillaries. Thus, even in exercise, where blood flow is increased, there is enough time for capillary O_2 and CO_2 to equilibrate with the alveolar air.

Although the pressure differences for CO_2 diffusion (only 45/40 between veins and alveoli, and 46/45 between cells and capillaries) are much less than that for

	pO$_2$	pCO$_2$
Atmospheric	159	0.3
Alveolar	104	40
Alveolar capillary	104	40
Arterial	95	40
Interstitial fluid	40	45
Intracellular	23	46
Venous	40	45

Figure 6-5

O$_2$ diffusion, CO$_2$ still diffuses well, since CO$_2$ intrinsically diffuses about 20 times more rapidly than O$_2$.

Apart from the measurement of blood gases, one may also evaluate respiratory effectiveness with **spirometry**, a technique for measuring respiratory effort. As the patient breathes in and out of the spirometer, the volume and time sequence is recorded as a graphic output.

Fig. 6-6. Terminology used in evaluating the respiratory effort:

TV—tidal volume
IRV—inspiratory reserve volume
ERV—expiratory reserve volume
RV—residual volume
FRC—functional residual capacity
IC—inspiratory capacity
VC—vital capacity
TLC—total lung capacity

Imagine a TV set (**TV**) in a house (the width of the house in the figure represents the difference in the volume of the lung between maximum inspiration and maximum expiration). On either side of the TV are Irving (**Irv**) and Erving (**Erv**). They get tired of the TV, so they go outside to use their **RV**. The weather is cold and icy, and they get into an accident, leading them to crash into their own house, whereupon they mutter "This frickin' ice!" (**FRC, IC**). They are admitted to the hospital where they have their vital signs (**VC**) taken. They recover because they are given tender loving care (**TLC**). Note that the terms higher up in the house are inclusive of the terms below them. The specific significance of each term is as follows:

Tidal volume (TV): the amount of air normally inhaled (or exhaled) with each average breath (about 500 ml when resting) like the steady tides going in and out. In exercise, the person acquires more oxygen at first by breathing more **deeply** (increasing tidal volume) and then, with more intense exercise, by increasing the respiratory **rate**. Interestingly, the cardiac response to exercise is in a sense similar, at first consisting largely of increased stroke volume, and then increased heart rate. As a result of these pulmonary and cardiac responses, the balance between alveolar ventilation and blood perfusion is maintained during exercise. With increased age, however, the maximum heart rate decreases.

Inspiratory reserve volume: the extra amount you could have inhaled after breathing in normally.

Expiratory reserve volume: the extra amount you could have exhaled after exhaling normally.

Residual volume: the residual left in the lung after the strongest expiration. If you didn't have a residual volume there would be marked fluctuations in CO$_2$ and O$_2$ content of blood passing through the lungs during respirations. After expiration, there would be no entry of O$_2$ into the blood stream or loss of CO$_2$.

Vital capacity (VC): a macho test of breathing capacity—the amount of air exchanged from the maximal intake to the most forceful expiration. There will be a decrease in vital capacity with diseases that decrease pulmonary compliance. The **compliance** of the respiratory system is the increase in chest volume with each degree of increase of alveolar pressure. The greater the increase in lung volume with a given increase in alveolar pressure, the greater the compliance.

$$\text{Compliance} = \Delta V / \Delta P$$

Compliance depends partly on the distensibility of the **lungs**, which can be impeded by pathology such as fibrosis, edema, and airway obstruction. Compliance also decreases with decreased distensibility of the **chest wall**, as may occur in kyphosis and scoliosis.

$$\text{Elastance} = \Delta P / \Delta V$$

Elastance is simply the reciprocal of compliance. It refers to the tendency of the respiratory system (or lung or chest wall separately) to spring back to its original shape after expansion. The greater the elastance (as may be found in pulmonary fibrosis, kyphosis, etc.), the greater the tendency to rebound, i.e. the greater the rise in pressure that results from an increase in lung volume.

For the lung, elastance is partly due to elastic tissue in the lungs, but is mainly due to surface tension produced by the fluid coating in the alveoli, which tends to resist expansion. This surface tension is normally kept at a reduced level by **surfactant,** a lipoprotein produced by the alveolar epithelium. In **hyaline membrane dis-**

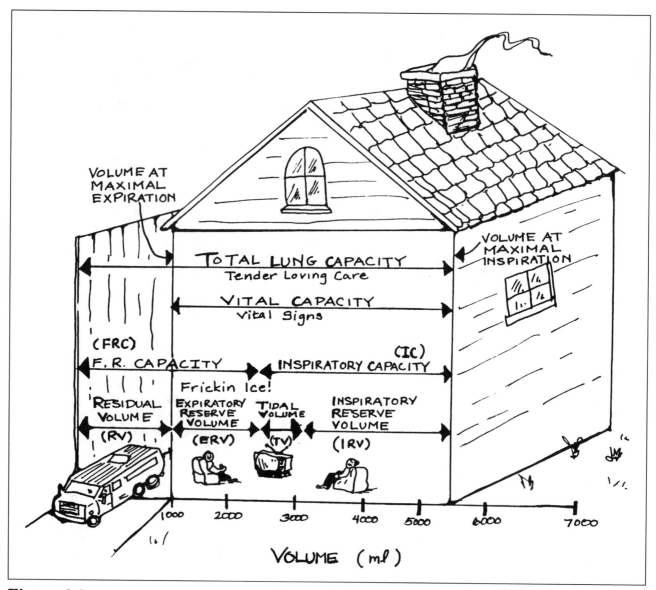

Figure 6-6

ease (**Infant Respiratory Distress Syndrome**), the newborn does not produce enough surfactant and hence the lungs cannot expand well due to the increased elastic resistance. The alveoli instead have a tendency to collapse (**atelectasis**).

Hypoxia in adults can also cause a loss of surfactant (either by decreasing its production or increasing its destruction), leading to **Adult Respiratory Distress Syndrome** ("**shock lung syndrome**"), with attendant atelectasis.

With increased elastic resistance, the work of breathing increases. The patient can try to compensate either by increasing the tidal volume or by breathing faster. When breathing difficulty is due to increased elasticity of the lungs or chest wall, the patient tends to compensate mainly by breathing faster, as it is too much work to deeply inspire. When it is resistance to flow that is increased, as occurs in the narrowing of the respiratory passages in asthma and chronic bronchitis, the patient often finds it less work to compensate by increasing the tidal volume rather than the rate. In fact, the rate of breathing may decrease.

Total lung capacity: the total amount of air in the lung after a forced inspiration.

Minute respiratory volume: the amount of air exchanged per minute. Minute respiratory volume = tidal volume (about 500 ml generally) × respiratory rate (about 12 breaths/min) = about 6 liters/min.

Dead space volume: the extra-alveolar area of the pulmonary tree (trachea and bronchial tree) in which no gas exchange occurs with the blood circulation. It is about 150 ml in adults.

Alveolar ventilation: the volume of fresh air entering the alveoli each minute. **Alveolar Ventilation** = Respiratory Rate × (Tidal Volume − Dead Space Volume). Alveolar ventilation is a particularly important clinical entity, as it, along with blood perfusion through the lungs, is critical in the exchange of gases between alveoli and blood.

One of the simplest ways to assess respiratory function is to have the patient inspire maximally to total lung capacity and then to expire fully as rapidly as possible. The total volume of the expired air (the **vital capacity**) is low in **restrictive lung disease**, where expansion of the lung is restricted (respiratory compliance is low; elastic rebound is high), e.g. pulmonary fibrosis. Vital capacity may also be low in **airway obstructive disease**, such as asthma, bronchitis, and emphysema; in those situations, the high intrapleural pressure of exhalation against the obstruction collapses the bronchial tree and reduces the amount that can be exhaled, leaving a lung with a high residual volume. (Vital capacity may also be decreased in a patient who does not cooperate for the test.)

The **rate** of expulsion of air (usually given as the amount expired in 1 second, or $FEV_{1.0}$) may be low in obstructive conditions like asthma, chronic bronchitis, emphysema, and tumors of the bronchial tree because of the obstructive factor. $FEV_{1.0}$ may also be decreased in restrictive lung disease, since the vital capacity is low and little air is expelled. (The degree of patient cooperation is also important in interpreting the test.)

An important distinction between obstructive and restrictive lung disease is that residual lung volume (RV) is increased in obstructive disease, but decreased in restrictive disease. Spirometry, however, cannot measure RV. Spirometry can measure tidal volume (TV), inspiratory reserve volume (IRV), and expiratory reserve volume (ERV) (as well as inspiratory capacity and vital capacity, which are combinations of TV, IRV and ERV). However, spirometry cannot measure RV (or functional residual capacity or total lung capacity, which require a knowledge of RV), simply because a patient cannot ex-

pire all the air in his/her lungs. To some qualitative degree residual volume can be assessed on the physical exam (barrel chest and resonant percussion may suggest increased residual volume) and on X-ray, but other tests are required for quantitative assessment. These include the nitrogen washout and helium-dilution methods, and body plethysmography, which are beyond the scope of this discussion.

Fig. 6-7. Differences between restrictive and obstructive disease.

In asthma, bronchitis, and emphysema, expiration is more difficult than inspiration, since the positive pressure of expiration collapses the respiratory passages. In fixed airway obstructions, there is difficulty with both inspiration and expiration. In upper airway (extrapulmonary) obstruction, inspiration may be more difficult than expiration since the negative pressure of inspiration is transmitted through the bronchi and trachea to cause constriction of areas higher up. (As an example, try breathing in while your cheeks are filled with air and your mouth and nose are closed. The cheeks will be sucked in.)

Treatment Of Respiratory Problems

Oxygen therapy (e.g. using an oxygen tent, face mask or nasal cannula) may be useful in hypoxia secondary to poor atmosphere oxygenation or to poor pulmonary gas exchange from lung disease. However, such therapy is not particularly useful in anemia or other disorders of blood cells, where there are either too few blood cells or impaired RBC function, since the extra O_2 does not drive much more O_2 into the blood. Oxygen also does not help where there is impaired tissue utilization of O_2, as in cyanide poisoning. Oxygen administration may help, though, in carbon monoxide poisoning. Carbon monoxide (CO) binds more strongly than does O_2 to the same site on the hemoglobin molecule, in effect reducing the number of available RBCs.

	RESTRICTIVE DISEASE	OBSTRUCTIVE DISEASE
Total Lung Capacity	↓	↑
Vital Capacity	↓	↓
$FEV_{1.0}$	↓	↓
Functional Residual Capacity	↓	↑

Figure 6-7

Treatment with pure oxygen or hyperbaric oxygen, can displace some CO by competition.

In administering oxygen for hypoxemic respiratory failure, it is important to avoid too high an oxygen concentration (the arterial pO_2 should be about 60mm Hg), since too high a pO_2 may decrease the patient's respiratory drive, and the patient's already elevated pCO_2 may rise even more, worsening the respiratory acidosis.

When the patient cannot breathe or the effort of breathing becomes too much for the patient, it may be necessary to use a mechanical ventilator. Normally, inspiration occurs because the chest expansion creates a **negative pressure** in the alveoli, which results in the influx of air from the atmosphere outside the patient, where the pressure is greater. It is possible to duplicate this by placing the patient's body, except for the head, in a chamber (**iron lung**) that rhythmically recreates the negative pressure.

More commonly, though, the ventilator is a **positive pressure** device that directly blows into the lungs air (or oxygen) that has greater than atmospheric pressure. There are a number of different modes of such ventilation. One format may deliver a set volume at periodic intervals, totally controlling the respiratory cycles for patients who are apneic (not breathing). In other modes the ventilator may assist the patient's weakened inspiratory efforts, responding when the patient inspires or at prolonged intervals between inspirations.

PEEP (positive end-expiratory pressure) is a form of positive pressure respiration that keeps the alveolar pressure above atmospheric pressure throughout the respiratory cycle, even after expiration. PEEP helps prevent alveolar collapse (atelectasis), as might otherwise occur, for instance, in the hypoxia-induced shock-lung syndrome, where there is a loss of pulmonary surfactant.

PART II: EVERYTHING ELSE

CHAPTER 7. BLOOD CELLS AND BLOOD COAGULATION

Pluripotential cells in the bone marrow differentiate into the major blood cells: red cells, white cells and platelets. The chapter on the immune system discusses the white cells.

Red Blood Cells

The major stimulus to red blood cell (RBC) production is **erythropoetin**, which is produced in the kidney. Anemia (a decrease in the number or concentration of red blood cells, or amount or concentration of hemoglobin) is a common inducer of erythropoetin production. It is not the number or concentration of RBCs that stimulates erythropoetin production, but decreased oxygenation of the blood. Thus, the number of red blood cells may increase in chronic hypoxia, such as occurs in those who live at high altitudes.

The effectiveness of the red blood cell in carrying oxygen depends on the oxygen supply, the number of red blood cells, and the health of the red cells:

1) In **aplastic anemia**, the marrow as a whole is suppressed, commonly by radiation or drugs. Red cells as well as other blood cells decrease in number (**pancytopenia**) in aplastic anemia.

2) Anemia can develop from significant **blood loss**.

3) If iron, an important ingredient of the hemoglobin molecule, is deficient in the diet, the patient develops an **iron deficiency anemia**. Iron is transported in the blood by a plasma protein, **transferrin**, and is stored intracellularly on another protein, **ferritin**. Deficiency of transferrin also results in an iron deficiency anemia.

4) Vitamin B_{12} and folic acid are important in the synthesis of DNA, especially in development of RBCs from their precursor cells in the marrow. A **deficiency of vitamin B_{12} or folic acid** will lead to a **megaloblastic anemia**, in which the RBCs are large, fragile, and short-lived.

Intrinsic factor, produced by parietal cells in the gastric mucosa, normally combines with vitamin B_{12}, protecting it from gastric digestion, and also facilitates its transport across the intestinal mucosal membrane. **Lack of intrinsic factor**, therefore, will also result in a megaloblastic anemia (pernicious anemia) due to failure of B_{12} absorption.

5) **Defects in the structure of hemoglobin** may be responsible for the anemia. For instance, in **sickle cell anemia**, a recessive gene results in abnormal hemoglobin, which distorts the red cells into a sickle shape in states of low oxygenation. The RBC becomes very fragile, is short-lived, and can clog blood vessels. About 8% of the black population carries the gene. Individuals with the heterozygous state typically are normal, although sickling can occur in marked states of hypoxia. True sickle cell anemia, the homozygous state, occurs in about 0.3% of blacks.

Unlike sickle cell anemia and many other hemoglobinopathies, the defect in the anemia of **thallasemia** is not due to a mutation that causes a single amino acid defect in the hemoglobin molecule. Rather, there is a defect in the **quantities** of particular polypeptide chains that are part of the hemoglobin molecule.

6) There may be **defects in the red cell membrane**, e.g. hereditary spherocytosis, hereditary elliptocytosis, and paroxysmal nocturnal hemoglobinuria.

7) There may be a **defect in the metabolic pathways** within red blood cells, e.g. pyruvate kinase deficiency and G6PD deficiency.

8) There may be an **immune reaction against red blood cells**, e.g. autoimmune processes or drug-related immune reactions. Any process that results in the premature destruction of red cells is termed a **hemolytic anemia.** Hemolytic anemias include those entities mentioned above in which there is an **intrinsic defect** in the red blood cell (membrane defects, metabolic defects, sickle cell anemia and other hemoglobinopathies). Also included are entities like immune reactions and infections, in which the attack on the RBCs originates **extrinsically.**

Platelets

Platelets are fragments of megakaryocyte cells, which originate in the bone marrow. Despite their small size (about 3 micrometers) platelets perform a number of functions important to the clotting process:

1) They stick to the damaged blood vessel wall, thereby participating in clot formation.

2) They contract, due to actin and myosin molecules within them, thereby facilitating clot retraction and closure of the damaged blood vessel.

3) They secrete **ADP** and **thromboxane A2**, which activate other platelets to become sticky and join in the clot-forming process.

4) **Platelet phospholipids** and **platelet factor 3** are important ingredients in the cascading pathway of blood clotting.

5) Platelets produce **fibrin-stabilizing factor**, which binds fibrin molecules into a meshwork and strengthens the clot.

6) Platelets produce **prostaglandins**, which have a number of different effects on blood flow and wound healing.

Blood Clotting

When a blood vessel is severed, a number of processes aid in wound closure:

1) Local constriction of the blood vessel, due to local neurogenic causes and local tissue chemical reactions.

2) Formation of a pure platelet plug, in the case of small wounds to capillaries or very small blood vessels. The pure platelet plug is often sufficient to close small wounds, even without a blood clot.

3) Formation of a blood clot, in the case of larger wounds. The blood clot contains not only platelets, but red blood cells and the reaction end products of the blood clotting processes, particularly fibrin.

4) Wound repair with formation of fibrous tissue.

Blood clotting involves a number of clotting factors:
Factor I (Fibrinogen)
Factor II (Prothrombin)
Factor III (Tissue thromboplastin)
Factor IV (Calcium)
Factor V (Proaccelerin)
Factor VII (Proconvertin)
Factor VIII (Antihemophilic factor A)
Factor IX (Antihemophilic factor B)
Factor X (Stuart factor)
Factor XI (Antihemophilic factor C)
Factor XII (Hageman factor)
HMW Kininogen (Fitzgerald factor)
Platelets
Prekallikrein (Fletcher factor)

Absence of a particular factor may lead to the failure of the clotting mechanism:

Fig. 7-1. The sequence of events in blood clotting:

1) Injury to the blood vessel wall or to the blood induces, after a number of steps, the formation of **prothrombin activator**.

2) Prothrombin activator catalyzes the change of **prothrombin to thrombin**.

3) Thrombin changes **fibrinogen to fibrin** threads, which mix with RBCs, platelets, and plasma to form a blood clot.

4) **Clot retraction**, assisted by platelets, expresses **serum** (serum is plasma minus its clotting factors, such as fibrinogen, etc). Plasma can clot. Serum cannot.

Sounds simple, huh? But what are the steps that lead to the formation of prothrombin activator? That is complex! There are an **extrinsic pathway** and an **intrinsic pathway**, both of which lead to the formation of prothrombin activator.

The extrinsic pathway is triggered by **tissue thromboplastin**, which is released from damaged cells in the vascular endothelial wall or outside the blood vessel.

The intrinsic pathway is triggered intrinsically by damage to the blood cells themselves, or by contact of the blood cells with a foreign surface, such as skin or collagen in the wound. A foreign surface also includes the glass in a blood collection tube. Hence, unless a collected blood specimen is mixed with an anticoagulant, it will clot in the glass tube due to activation of the intrinsic pathway.

Both the intrinsic and extrinsic pathways involve a number of clotting factor enzymes which participate in cascading reactions that ultimately lead to the formation of prothrombin activator.

Fig. 7-1 shows a simplified schema of the ingredients of the intrinsic and extrinsic cascading pathways of blood clotting. The extrinsic pathway normally occurs quite quickly; blood may clot within 15 seconds of activation of the extrinsic pathway. Clotting takes a number of minutes, however, along the intrinsic pathway, which has more steps than the extrinsic pathway.

Clinical Disorders of Clotting

1) The normal platelet count is >150,000 per microliter. If the count falls below 50,000 (**thrombocytopenia**), the patient develops numerous widespread dot-like (**petechial**) hemorrhages and is at great risk for a major life-threatening hemorrhage. The causes include bone marrow depression, immune disorders, and various infections.

Von Willebrandt's disease is a hemorrhagic disease in where there is a defect in the adhesion of platelets to the subendothelial collagen in the capillary wall. The bleeding time is prolonged. Aspirin also prolongs the bleeding time as it decreases platelet adhesivity.

2) Factor VIII is missing in the most common **hemophilia** (Hemophilia A, or classic hemophilia—about 85% of the hemophilias), and Factor IX is missing in the remainder (Hemophilia B—about 15%). Hemophilia is a rare disorder of bleeding that is carried as an X-linked recessive gene. Therefore, the disease is es-

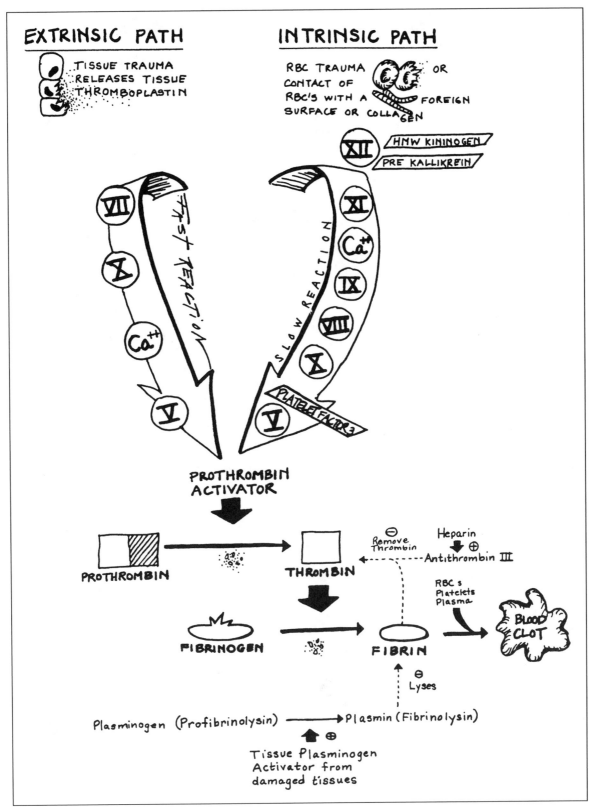

Figure 7-1

sentially a male disorder, and classic hemophilia affects about one in 10,000 males in the U.S. Males with one hemophilia gene develop hemophilia, whereas females with one hemophilia gene are carriers.

3) Calcium (Factor IV) is important to the clotting process, but does not decrease enough to present a clinical clotting problem. However, substances are commonly added to collected blood samples to remove calcium from the blood and prevent the blood from clotting in the tube (e.g. citrate or oxalate ions)

4) Severe liver disease, such as cirrhosis and hepatitis, can cause clotting problems, since most of the clotting factors are produced by the liver (e.g. prothrombin, fibrinogen, etc.).

5) Deficiency of vitamin K may cause bleeding problems, because vitamin K is important in the formation of prothrombin and factors VII, IX, and X. Normally, we get plenty of vitamin K in the diet, and it is also produced by bacteria in the gut, but in conditions of fat malabsorption (vitamin K is a fat-soluble vitamin), vitamin K deficiency may occur.

The body normally has a number of negative feedback mechanisms that prevent clotting from proceeding excessively:

1) Fibrin in the clot absorbs excess thrombin.

2) A globulin in the clot area called anti-thrombin III inactivates excess thrombin.

3) **Heparin**, a powerful anticoagulant produced by mast cells and basophils, enhances the activity of antithrombin III. Heparin is commonly used clinically as an anticoagulant. It has immediate anticoagulant effects. It is administered intravenously. **Coumarin** is another clinically used anticoagulant, which acts by a different mechanism. It competes with vitamin K and inhibits the production in the liver of prothrombin and other clotting factors. It is given orally, but requires one or more days to take effect, since one must wait for the existing prothrombin to be depleted.

4) Plasma contains a protein called **plasminogen (profibrinolysin)**, which, when activated, becomes **plasmin (fibrinolysin)**. Fibrinolysin lyses fibrin and helps remove the clot. The process of plasminogen activation is relatively slow, occurring at least a day after the clot has formed to allow time for the initation of wound healing. It is activated by **tissue plasminogen activator**, which is released by the damaged tissues.

Coagulation Tests

Tests for the integrity of the coagulation mechanism are based on whether one wishes to test the intrinsic or extrinsic pathway, or platelet function, as follows:

1) Tests of the intrinsic pathway: The **whole blood clotting time** test measures the time taken for blood to clot in a glass test tube (normally about 9–15 minutes). This tests the intrinsic pathway, which is activated by contact with a foreign surface. If any component of the intrinsic pathway is defective, the clotting time will be prolonged over normal controls. One can then identify the particular component that is defective by assaying for particular clotting factors.

The **partial thromboplastin time (PTT)**, like the whole blood clotting time, tests for the integrity of the intrinsic pathway. Clotting in a test tube is initially prevented by citrating the plasma to remove calcium. The PTT measures the time taken for recalcified citrated plasma to clot in the test tube.

2) Tests of the extrinsic pathway: The one step **prothrombin time (PT)** is the time needed for recalcified citrated plasma to clot in the presence of tissue thromboplastin. Thus, the "protime" adds the critical tissue ingredient (tissue thromboplastin) that is necessary to start off the relatively fast extrinsic pathway. The normal protime is about 11–15 seconds. If the protime is prolonged, in relation to controls, this suggests a problem somewhere in the extrinsic pathway. **Mnemonic**: PTT (the test for the intrinsic path) has more letters than PT (the test for the extrinsic path), corresponding to the intrinsic path having more steps than the extrinsic path.

3) Tests of platelet function. Platelet function may be diminished either because of decreased numbers of platelets or because of a deficiency in the functioning of existing platelets.

A **platelet count** is, of course, useful in assessing the number of platelets. Bleeding may occur with low platelet counts. The **bleeding time** assesses platelet function. A small cut is placed on the patient's forearm, with a blood pressure cuff kept on the arm at 40mm Hg to resist venous flow. Normal bleeding time (depending on method) may be 2–7 min. Bleeding time tends to be normal in coagulation disorders of the extrinsic and intrinsic pathways, because the platelet plug operates independently of these pathways and is sufficient in itself to close up such small wounds. If the bleeding time is prolonged, this usually suggests a defect in platelet function.

The examination of both PTT and PT tests is useful to distinguish extrinsic from intrinsic coagulation disorders:

	PT	*PTT*
Intrinsic path defect	Normal	Abnormal
Extrinsic path defect	Abnormal	Normal
Liver failure, vitamin K deficiency, coumarin or heparin therapy	Abnormal	Abnormal

Neither the intrinsic nor extrinsic pathway can cause clotting if there is a defect at the end steps of prothrombin to thrombin or fibrinogen to fibrin. Therefore, both the prothrombin time and PTT will be abnormal in severe liver disease (the liver manufactures prothrombin, fibrinogen and other clotting factors), vitamin K deficiency, (vitamin K is necessary for formation of prothrombin and other factors), coumarin therapy (coumarin interferes with the formation of prothrombin and other clotting factors), and heparin administration (heparin indirectly inactivates thrombin).

CHAPTER 8.   THE IMMUNE SYSTEM.

The main function of the immune system is protection from foreign organisms and substances. Its key strategy is to distinguish self from non-self, and to eliminate the foreign. An **antigen** is any substance (usually foreign) that can combine with an antibody specific for it. **Antibodies** are immunoglobulin proteins that combine with (usually) foreign molecules (the antigens) and are specific for the particular antigen.

Although much attention has focused on highly specific defense molecules, such as antibodies, much defense occurs through less specific mechanisms that arose prior to the time that antibodies evolved, and which still persist today as vital components of the specific immune response. These less specific mechanisms are called **natural immunity**, as opposed to the more specific **adaptive immunity** of antibodies and like molecules.

Fig. 8-1. Actors in the immune response

Natural immunity, apart from obvious mechanisms such as stomach acidity and the physical barrier of the skin, include a diversity of molecules and cell types:

Molecules Of Natural Immunity

Interferon: a group of glycoproteins that, among other things, kills **viruses** and in general activates macrophages to do a better job in killing phagocytosed microorganisms. Most cells can secrete interferon, an important cellular defense mechanism, considering that viruses must live within cells.

Lysozyme: a natural antibiotic against **bacteria** that is produced by macrophages and neutrophils, and which attacks the bacterial cell wall.

Complement: includes at least 15 proteins, mostly enzyme precursors, which are produced in part in the liver, found in the serum, and, when **activated**, un-

ACTORS IN THE IMMUNE RESPONSE			
Natural Immunity		Adaptive Immunity	
Molecules	Cells	Molecules	Cells
Interferon	Macrophages	Antibodies	B lymphocytes
Lysozyme	Microglia		T lymphocytes
Complement	Dendritic cells		T-helper cells
C-reactive protein	Langerhans cells		T-cytolytic cells
Prostaglandins	Kupffer cells		T-suppressor
Kinins	Alveolar macrophages		cells
Leukotrienes and	Neutrophils		
other cytokines	Eosinophils		
	Basophils		
	Mast cells		
	Platelets		
	Natural killer cells		
	Vascular endothelial cells		
	Kidney mesangial cells		
	Reticular cells		

Figure 8-1

dergo cascading chain reaction conversions that are important in the immune response.

In the **classical pathway** of complement activation, the factor that activates complement is an antigen-antibody complex. In the **alternative pathway**, complment activation does not require interaction of complement with an antigen/antibody complex. Rather, bacterial lipopolysaccharide (LPS, endotoxin) and other general bacterial substances (also immunoglobulin A aggregates) can activate complement. In both the classical and alternative pathways, a key outcome is the conversion of the C3 component of complement into C3a and C3b proteins. These different forms of complement have different functions:

Fig. 8-2. Functions of complement. The Complement Can is spilling "OIL" (Opsonization, Inflammation, Lysis).

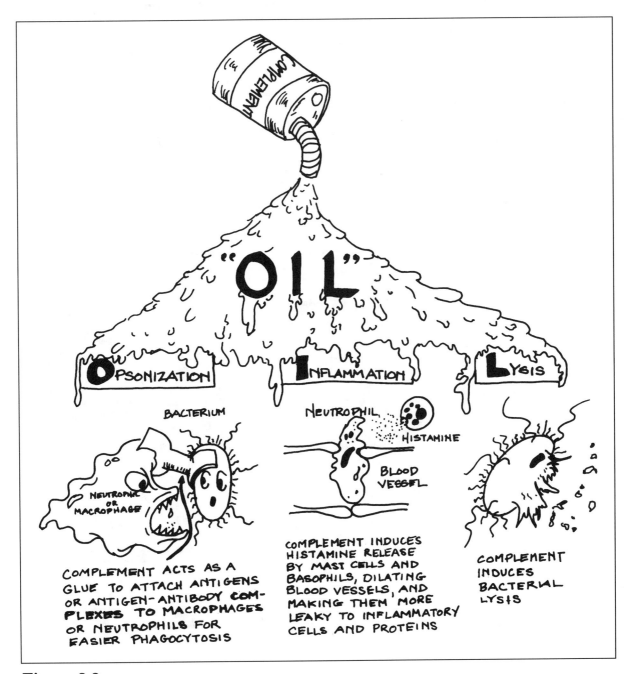

Figure 8-2

1) **Opsonization** (C3b) is a "gluing" process that attaches bacteria to neutrophils and macrophages, which then can more readily eat (**phagocytose**) them. (**Mnemonic**: C,3, and b "stick" together as all the letters rhyme.) Opsonization is particularly important to attach the tough-to-attack encapsulated bacteria to phagocytic cells.

Although complement does not act with the specificity of antibodies, it does indirectly participate in the specific elimination of antibody/antigen complexes by attaching such complexes to phagocytic cells, which then can eliminate them more efficiently. Complement may also remove immune complexes by attaching the antigen-antibody complexes to red cells, which drop off the complexes in the liver and spleen for removal. Complement may directly deal with bacteria and viruses by promoting bacterial agglutination and neutralizing the virulence of certain viruses. Complement may also prevent antigen/antigen complexes from forming in the first place, which may be useful in situations where deposition of an antigen/antibody complex may prove harmful.

2) **Inflammation.** Other forms of complement (e.g. C3a) can stimulate an acute inflammatory response,

inducing histamine release from mast cells and basophils. This renders blood vessels more leaky so that neutrophils and other inflammatory cells, as well as complement protein, can enter the damaged tissue. Certain complement components may in themselves exert a **chemotactic** (chemical attraction) influence on neutrophils.

The general inflammatory response is complex, including as its goal not only the defeat of invading organisms, but wound healing as well. Scavenger cells, such as macrophages and neutrophils, not only take care of invading organisms, but also clean up damaged tissue. Intertwined with the antibiotic effect of the immune system are clotting mechanisms, which stop bleeding, with the formation of fibrin, into which fibroblasts migrate and produce collagen, which helps form a healing scar.

Fig. 8-3. The inflammatory response. Symptoms are calor (heat), rubor (redness), tumor (swelling), dolor (pain) and functio laesa (loss of function).

3) **Lysis**. Certain forms of activated complement can bore their way through the cell walls of bacteria and destroy them through cell leakage (lysis).

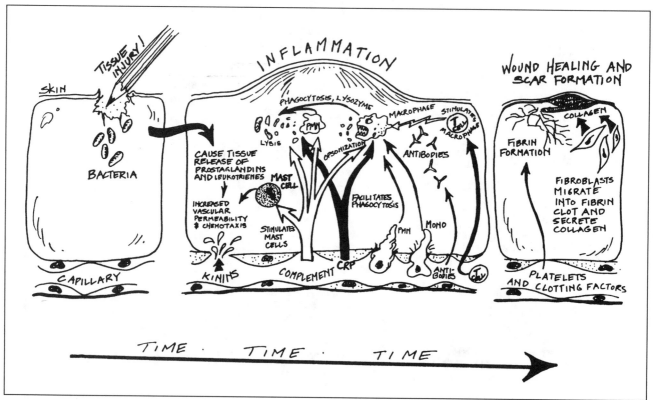

Figure 8-3

C-reactive protein: a type of serum globulin that is produced in the liver and increases during acute tissue injury or inflammation. It binds to the surface of bacteria and facilitates phagocytosis. The acute phase of inflammation can often be detected in the laboratory through measurement of C-reactive protein.

Prostaglandins and **leukotrienes:** fatty acids that may be released by damaged cells, including mast cells. They have a variety of functions, such as enhancement of the inflammatory response by increasing vascular permeability, chemotaxis (chemical attraction) of neutrophils toward the wound site, and stimulating pain endings.

Kinins: serum proteins that stimulate vascular dilation and permeability during inflammatory reactions.

Interleukins. Among other things, interleukins stimulate the proliferation and maturation of lymphocytes during the immune response.

Colony-stimulating factors (CSFs). Among other things, CSFs stimulate the proliferation and development of granulocytes, monocytes and macrophages. **Erythropoetin** is a CSF that is produced in the kidney and stimulates red cell production.

Tumor Necrosis Factors (TNF). Among other things, TNF can attack tumors by damaging their blood vessels.

TGF-beta. Among other things, TGF-beta can inhibit a variety of cytokines.

Cytokine is a general term, usually signifying a protein hormone that affects the function of cells lying near the cell of origin of the cytokine. A cytokine produced by a lymphocyte is called a **lymphokine**, whereas a cytokine produced by a mononuclear phagocyte (macrophage) is called a **monokine.** This discussion, for simplicity, will use the general term "cytokine." A number of the above-mentioned molecules are cytokines, including interleukins, interferons, colony-stimulating factors, tumor necrosis factors, and TGF-beta. The many kinds of cytokines often overlap in their functions.

Cells Of Natural Immunity

Fig. 8-4. Cell lineage in the immune system.

Monocytes, which are found in the blood, are the precursors of tissue macrophages, which participate in natural immunity. The various kinds of tissue phagocytic cells include:

1) **Macrophages.** Macrophages, without the assistance of antibodies, can often recognize and directly phagocytose many kinds of bacteria, in addition to recognizing and cleaning up damaged tissues Macrophages can also kill many bacteria without phagocytosing them, by secreting toxic enzymes, e.g. **lysozyme.** The Golgi apparatus inside macrophages spins off **lysosomes**, which contain lysozyme and other digestive enzymes that are either secreted or used internally to digest bacteria. For internal digestion, the lysosome fuses with a **phagosome** (a vesicle containing a phagocytosed microorga ism) to form a **phagolysosome**, where the microorganism is killed and digested internally.

Fig. 8-5. Action of lysozyme either externally or internally to kill bacteria.

Fig. 8-6. A granuloma. In chronic inflammation, macrophages may move together to form a **granuloma**, another means of defense. Granulomas contain **epithelioid cells** (macrophages that have acquired a large amount of cytoplasm) and **multinucleated giant cells** (a fusion of a number of macrophage cells). Fibrosis with calcification frequently occurs around granulomas. Granulomas wall off infectious material from the rest of the body. They may form if the phagocytic cells cannot digest the foreign material (e.g. asbestos, silica). Indigestible immune complexes may also induce granulomas. Granulomas also arise when there is a continuing irritant stimulus. Thus, granulomas may form in certain autoimmune diseases, where there is a persistent reaction to the host's antigens.

2) **Microglia**, phagocytic cells found in the brain.

3) **Dendritic cells**, found in the spleen and lymph nodes, play an important role in presenting antigen to lymphocytes (discussed later).

4) **Langerhans cells**, found in the skin, are weakly phagocytic cells that are important in presenting antigen to lymphocytes.

5) **Kupffer cells**, phagocytic cells found within blood sinus walls in the liver.

6) **Alveolar macrophages**, found in the lung.

The above-mentioned phagocytic cells are collectively termed the "**reticulo-endothelial system**" (the term does not include the neutrophil).

T helper lymphocytes (discussed later) need to be properly introduced to antigen in order for them to react to the antigen; the antigen generally needs to be presented to the T helper cell by another cell. A number of phagocytic cells (particularly macrophages, dendritic cells, and Langerhans cells) not only are phagocytic but also present antigens to T lymphocytes. (Endothelial cells and B lymphocytes can also present antigens to T cells.)

Note that stem cells in the bone marrow give rise to monocytes, which in turn give rise to the above-

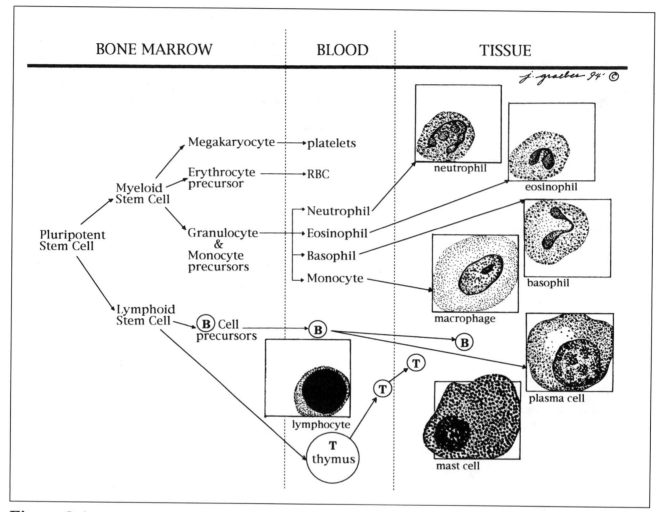

Figure 8-4

mentioned categories of phagocytic cells. Bone marrow cells also give rise to **granulocytes** (neutrophils, eosinophils, and basophils, which contain visible granules) and **platelets**:

Neutrophils are scavenger white cells. These short-lived cells (living only up to 1–2 days) quickly exit the blood stream into inflamed tissues. (Lymphocytes and monocytes arrive last.) Neutrophil granules contain potent bacteriocidal enzymes used for internal digestion of bacteria.

Eosinophils increase in number in parasitic, notably worm, infestation. They contain cell surface receptors for immunoglobulin E (IgE), which is produced at high levels in parasitic infection. In response to antigens that attach to eosinophil cell-bound IgE, eosinophilic cell granules release substances that are toxic to parasitic worms, which often are resistant to

neutrophil and macrophage lysozymes. Eosinophils also increase in number during allergic reactions in which there is stimulation of IgE production, but their function in allergic hypersensitivity is not clear. Like neutrophils, eosinophils can exit through blood vessel walls into the tissues.

Basophils are granulated white cells in the blood that also can exit the blood stream into the tissues. Their granules contain heparin and vasoactive amines, such as histamine and 5-hydroxytryptamine, which increase vascular permeability and allow inflammatory cells and complement to enter the tissues from the blood stream.

Mast cells, unlike the circulating basophils, are not found in the blood. They are tissue-based, but are believed to mature in the tissues from immature precursor cells from the bone marrow. Like basophils, their

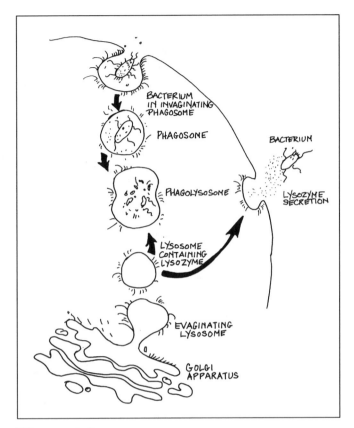

Figure 8-5

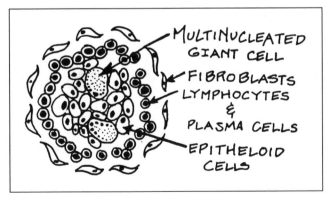

Figure 8-6

granules contain powerful inflammatory substances (e.g. histamine, 5-hydroxytryptamine) which, when secreted, increase vascular permeability and allow inflammatory cells and complement to enter the tissues from the blood stream. Both basophils and mast cells have surface IgE receptors. Secretion occurs when antigen binds to cell-bound IgE on basophils and mast cells.

Unlike the granulocytes, it is believed that mast cells do not originate in the bone marrow.

Platelets, although usually considered in the context of blood clotting, platelets can also phagocytose antigen/antibody complexes.

Natural killer cells are lymphocyte-like cells that can kill virus-containing cells, but do so without the high-specificity characteristics of the B and T lymphocytes.

There are other kinds of phagocytic cells that arise not from bone marrow stem cells, but from the tissue mesenchyme throughout the body. These include:

Vascular endothelial cells, which can produce and respond to lymphokines, and present antigen to lymphocytes.

Bone osteoclast cells, which resorb bone.

Kidney mesangium cells in the renal glomeruli, which can phagocytose antigen/antibody complexes that deposit there.

71

Reticular cells of the lymph nodes, spleen, thymus and bone marrow.

Adaptive Immunity

As higher animals evolved, invading organisms also evolved and developed defense mechanisms against the simple natural immunity of the human host. Faced with the difficulty of defending against the rapid mutations of bacteria, viruses, and other organisms, the more advanced organisms decided on the strategy of developing specific antibodies against **all** possible antigens.

Antibodies are produced by **plasma cells**, which are derived from **B lymphocytes**. Antibody production constitutes **humoral immunity**. Another form of adaptive immunity, **cell-mediated immunity**, requires direct contact of the antigen with lymphocytes, notably **T lymphocytes**, and is not mediated through antibodies.

Antibodies and B Cells

Fig. 8-7. Structure of the IgG antibody molecule. The myriad specificities of the antibodies are determined by the variable portions of the antibody molecule, which re-

side in the Fab portions of the molecule. There are two Fab sections—the two arms of the "Y," each of which contains a heavy and a light chain. The variable portion (V) is at the free end of each Fab segment arm. The rest of the molecule is constant (C) in all the IgG molecules of the individual.

An antigen must be a macromolecule, either a large protein or polysaccharide, in order to activate lymphocytes to generate antibody formation. If an antigen is too small to generate an immune response by itself, it is called a **hapten**. If it is large enough to generate an immune response, it is called an **immunogen**. The areas on immunogens on which antigens reside are called **determinants,** or **epitopes.** A large immunogen may have many epitopes. Semantically, epitopes are really haptens attached to a macromolecule.

Fig. 8-8. The structure and function of the major antibody groups, or **isotypes**. A mnemonic for the various isotypes is "GAMED"—immunoglobulins G, A, M, E, and D, or IgG, IgA, IgM, IgE, and IgD. The particular isotype is determined by the constant, Fc (**Fraction "c"**) portion. **IgG** is the main, classic immunoglobulin. **IgA** is the main antibody in secretions and plays a significant role in first-line defense at the mucosal level. **IgM** is the main antibody in the initial "primary" immune response and shows good complement activation in view of its large ("**Magnum**") size, consisting of five IgG-like subunits. **IgE** is found in allergy and worm infestation. Its Fc region binds to eosinophils, basophils and mast cells and is a significant mediator of allergic hypersensitivity reactions when antigen binds to surface-bound IgE. **IgD** is an antigen receptor on B lymphocytes. (It is not the only antigen receptor, however. IgM can also be an antigen receptor on primary lymphocytes, whereas IgG, IgA, and IgE can be antigen receptors on "memory" lymphocytes, those lymphocytes which respond the second time around to antigen stimulation.)

It was no small evolutionary task to develop as many as a billion different antibodies against all possible antigens, considering the limited number of genes in the human genome. According to the **clonal selection theory**, the human immune system, prior to any antigen stimulation, already contains numerous clones of antibody-producing cells, each different clone confined to producing only one specific antibody for one specific antigen. The immune system, thus, prior to being introduced to foreign antigens, already contains the antibody repertoire against all of them. In addition to the enormous amount of information necessary to create such a repertoire, such a strategy had to result in antibodies against only foreign antigens, while leaving the host cell antigens intact.

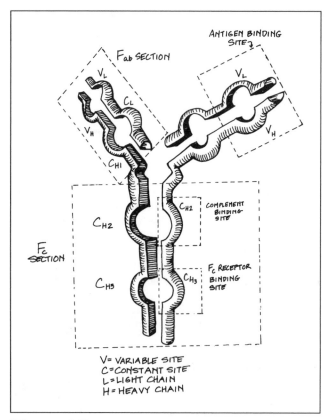

Figure 8-7

Immunoglobulin	Structure	Function
IgG	monomer	prominent in secondary response
IgA	dimer	prominent in secretions
IgM	pentamer	prominent in antibody response
IgE	long Fc fragment	prominent in worm infestations & allergies. Binds to Fc receptors on mast cells and basophils causing them to release inflammatory substances
IgD	?	receptor on B-lymphocytes

Figure 8-8

The body resolved the problem of this enormous information requirement in much the same way as one obtains card combinations in a shuffled deck. A single deck contains 52 cards. If each card represented a single gene for a single antibody, one could obtain only 52 antibodies. However, if an antibody consists of a combination of one club, one spade, one heart, and one diamond, each suit reflecting a different gene for a segment of the antibody molecule, then the number of combinations is vastly increased. The variable portions of the heavy and light chains of the antibody molecule are each formed by such a mechanism: the subdivisions of each variable portion are formed independently and shuffled to produce many different variable segments. The combination of a variable portion of a heavy chain with a variable portion of a light chain compounds the possibilities. Mutations can also increase the variations. In addition, there are the five antibody isotypes (GAMED),

which are determined by the constant portion of the antibody molecule. Thus the number of kinds of antibody molecules is compounded by the association of the myriad variable portions with any of the five basic constant portions.

Allotopes are inherited small, functionally insignificant, structural differences, especially in the constant portion of the antibody molecule, that differentiate an isotype of one individual from that of another. In a given individual (and the individual's identical twin), all the molecules of a given isotype belong to the same allotope.

In the end, only one specific antibody is produced by each antibody-producing B lymphocyte. **Monoclonal antibodies** are identical antibody molecules synthesized by a clone of cells that arose from a single antibody-producing cell. Monoclonal antibodies may be created in tissue culture conditions, but may also be found in certain lymphocytic tumors. Monoclonal antibody formation is not, however, the typical response in vivo to a single antigenic stimulus. What usually occurs is that a single antigen stimulates a variety of closely related lymphocytes to produce different antibodies that more or less resemble the correct fit for the antigen. (Each of those antibodies may attack different antigens that more or less resemble one another.) The subsequent rise in plasma antibody on an electrophoresis analysis is then broader than a single sharp spike.

It is important for the immune mechanism to distinguish self from non-self to avoid adverse interaction with the individual's own cells. One mechanism of such **self-tolerance** of B or T cells is the elimination, or inactivation, of those B and T cells that interact with self antigens. Such elimination is believed to occur during fetal development, but also in later life as immature lymphocytes arise. It appears that a given immature B or T cell interacts with its corresponding self-antigen, leading to the death, or at least inactivation, of the self-reactive lymphocyte. The exact mechanism is still unclear, but it is believed that self-reactive T lymphocytes are eliminated in the thymus gland, where T cells mature under the influence of thymic hormones.

The key cell responsible for adaptive immunity is the lymphocyte, each of which specifically can act against only one particular antigen. The specific lymphocytes include B cells and T cells:

B cell lymphocytes originate in the **B**one marrow. They **B**low out free-floating anti**B**odies into the **B**loodstream. (Actually, it is the plasma cell, derived from the B cell, that produces the antibody.) When an antigen contacts a matched B cell, it stimulates the specific surface immunoglobulin on the B cell, which in turn stimulates the B cell to divide and form plasma cells and B memory cells:

Plasma cells produce the specific antibody against the antigen. Contrary to the name, few plasma cells are found in the plasma. Most reside in lymphatic tissue, particularly the lymph nodes and the spleen. The secreted antibody enters the bloodstream, though. **Humoral immunity**, as mentioned, refers to immunity based on B cell generation of circulating antibody, in contrast to **cell-mediated immunity**, which requires direct contact of the antigen with lymphocytes, particularly T cells.

In general, **protein** antigens can generate both primary and secondary responses of antibody production. The **primary response** is the antibody production after first-time exposure to an antigen. It commonly requires 5–10 days and has relatively low production of antibody, mainly of the IgM type, as opposed to the IgG type.

The **secondary response**, which occurs with the second exposure to the antigen, is quicker (1–3 days) and produces a greater amount of antibody, mainly the IgG type (sometimes IgA or IgE). The major reason for the enhanced secondary response is the proliferation of **B memory cells** during the primary response. The secondary response is also much more specific for the particular offending antigen than is the primary response, a phenomenon termed **affinity maturation**.

Although protein antigens ultimately result in the production of antibodies, and antibodies are produced by plasma cells, which are B cell derivatives, T helper cells are necessary for this process, because T helper cells facilitate B memory cell proliferation and differentiation into plasma cells.

Carbohydrate antigen can stimulate a primary response, but they do not stimulate an enhanced secondary response. This is so because carbohydrate antigens do not act on T cells and thus, without the help of T cells, do not result in the production of memory cells. Thus, carbohydrate-induced immune responses tend to be shorter lived than protein-induced immune responses.

Idiotypes are the specific antigen receptors on B or T cells that distinguish the numerous lymphocytes from another. On B cells, the receptor is identical to the antibody produced by the B cell. On T cells, which do not produce antibodies, the receptors are very different, but still have amino acid sequences that partially resemble those of antibodies. The inducement of memory cells by protein antigens is a good reason for development of **antiidiotype vaccines**, instead of immunization by the corresponding carbohydrate antigen. An antibody against a host idiotype has the same key determinant **shape** as a corresponding carbohydrate antigen that fits into the same host antibody; such an antiidiotype antibody may therefore be useful for immunization, because, being a protein, it will induce memory cell proliferation and a stronger immunogenic response against the antigen.

B memory cells are an expanded population of B cells that originate in an immune response and enable a quicker response to the same antigen in the future. B memory cells originate in lymphoid tissue germinal centers. They then circulate in the blood to establish positions in more distant body areas. (T helper cells also form memory cells, but their location is less clear.)

B lymphocytes can respond either to free-floating antigens or to antigens on other cells. Macrophages and other kinds of accessory cells (e.g. dendritic cells) release interleukin-1 (IL-1), which stimulates T helper cells, which in turn produce cytokines that stimulate the proliferation and conversion of B lymphocytes to plasma and memory cells. Thus, the combination of antigen, cytokines from macrophages or other accessory cells, and cytokines from the T helper cells induces B cell proliferation.

Fig. 8-9. T helper cell function.

T cell lymphocytes originate in the **Thymus**. Rather than produce antibody, T cells contain cell-surface antibody-like molecules with which the T cell directly **Touches** the antigen (so called "cell-mediated" immunity). The antigen generally is presented to the T cell by another cell, such as a macrophage, spleen or lymph node dendritic cell, skin Langerhans cell, vascular endothelial cell, or B cell. Cell-mediated immunity differs from humoral immunity (the circulating antibody immunity of B cells) in that humoral antibody can be transferred from donor to host via cell-free plasma. Cell-mediated immunity, though, can only be transferred via T cells. In general, free-floating antigens are dealt with through free-floating antibodies, whereas intracellular organisms, like viruses and certain bacteria, which cannot be reached by antibodies, are dealt with best through cell-mediated immunity, in which the cell containing the microbe is attacked. Both cell-mediated immunity and the antibodies of humoral immunity can act on antigens affixed to cell surfaces.

There are several kinds of T cells: T helper cells (Th), T cytotoxic cells (Tc), and T suppressor cells:

1) **T helper cells (Th).** When antigen presentation activates a Th cell, the Th cell secretes cytokines that stimulate B cell proliferation and antibody production. Not all B cells, though, require interaction with Th cells in order to produce antibodies.

Th cells are particularly sophisticated cells. In order to respond to the antigen in the first place, the antigen not only has to be properly introduced to the Th cell through another cell (commonly a macrophage, lymphoid tissue dendritic cell, skin Langerhans cell, vascular endothelial cell, or a B lymphocyte), but the etiquette of the introduction requires that the presenting cell be recognized as a member of the host's family, namely as a host cell, as evidenced by the presence on the presenting cell of a **major histocompatibility complex (MHC, also called HLA, or "Human Leukocyte Antigen")** that is common to the cells of the host. The MHC, while not an antibody, contains a number of amino acid sequences that resemble those in antibodies and render the cells of a particular host unique to the individual. Identical twins, though, have the identical MHC.

The receptor on the T helper cell thus is responsive to the combination of antigen and host-matching MHC complex on the presenting cell. In general, the presenting cell first phagocytoses the protein antigen and cleaves it to peptides in the presenting cell's lysosomes before extruding the modified (peptide) antigen, which attaches to the presenting cell's surface MHC complex. The presenting cell, in addition to presenting the antigen, **also** releases IL-1, which induces T helper cell proliferation (see Fig. 8-9). The T helper cell that has been affected by IL-1, produces IL-2 and other cytokines, which in turn stimulate still further T cell proliferation and B cell proliferation and differentiation into plasma cells (Fig. 8-9). Like B cell proliferation, T cell proliferation results in memory cells, but of the T cell variety. B and T memory cells can persist a lifetime.

The MHC on the antigen-presenting cell, in the normal immune response, is a specific type called MHC II. MHC II is mainly found on macrophages and B lymphocytes, as well as dendritic cells and Langerhans cells. Another form of MHC, MHC I, is found more diffusely, on many kinds of cells. Both MHC I and MHC II are important in graft rejection. Th cells interact with those graft cells that contain MHC II receptors, whereas cytotoxic T cells (described below) interact with, and kill, the broad variety of foreign graft cells that contain MHC I receptors. Graft rejection may also be mediated through production of host antibodies against the graft.

It is believed that the particular MHC that an individual has may relate to the probability of developing particular autoimmune diseases.

T helper cells are quite "helpful." In addition to stimulating proliferation of B cells, T helper cells and T cytotoxic cells (discussed below), T helper cells also facilitate the removal of bacteria in still another way. Sometimes bacteria, although phagocytosed by macrophages, are not killed by the phagocytosing cells. Certain T helper cells, on recognizing bacterial antigen (in conjunction with MHC II complex) on the surface of the bacteria-filled macrophage, secrete cytokines that stimulate the macrophage (**macrophage activating factor; MAF**) to lyse the phagocytosed bacteria intracellularly as well as produce macrophage factors that kill bacteria extracellularly. T helper cells also produce macrophage **migration inhibition factor (MIF)**, which keeps macrophages in the general vicinity of the T helper cell. Cytokines are interesting in that they do not exhibit specificity for any particular bacterial or viral antigen, but nonetheless are an integral part of the specific immune response through their interaction with specific kinds of immune cells.

T helper cells also respond to foreign MHCs, such as might be introduced in a graft. Apparently, the T helper cells regard the foreign MHC as a "host MHC + antigen" combination and respond by stimulating T cytotoxic cells (see below), B cells and macrophages to attack

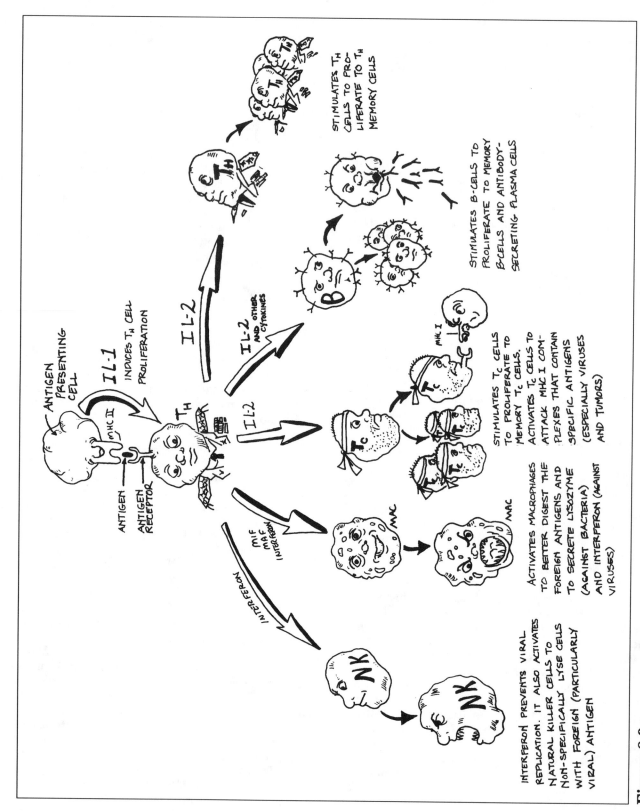

Figure 8-9

foreign cells. The MHC thus is an important factor in transplantation rejection.

2) **Cytotoxic T cells.** When antigen is presented to a B cell, the B cell attacks the antigen by converting into a plasma cell, which in turn produces antibody against the antigen. Cytotoxic T cells attack the antigen differently. The T cytotoxic cell is mainly concerned with defense against viruses, which are intracellular. It kills the cell that hosts the virus. Instead of producing antibody, the T cytotoxic cell directly combines with the degraded virus peptide antigen (previously degraded intracellularly), which is attached to the host's MHC I complex on the surface of the infected cell. In the case of graft rejection, the T cytotoxic cell considers the foreign MHC I (which is present on a wide variety of cells) to be a "host cell + virus" combination, and widely destroys the grafted cells.

3) **T suppressor cells** suppress both B and T cells and provide an important negative feedback mechanism in the immune response, ensuring that the immune response is not excessive and harmful to the individual. Probably the most important negative feedback mechanism in the immune system, though, is simply the disappearance of antigen during the course of the immune response. With no antigen, there is no immune reaction to antigen.

The treatment of maternal **Rh incompatibility** is an example of a feedback mechanism that eliminates the offending antigen. An Rh negative mother, by definition, carries no Rh red cell antigens. If the fetus is Rh positive, then at the time of gestation, and delivery in particular, some fetal cells enter the maternal blood stream and can stimulate antibody formation against the red cells. Such antibodies can damage the fetus in subsequent deliveries. In order to prevent this, the mother is administered anti-Rh factor antibody right after the first delivery. This antibody combines with the fetal antigen and prevents the antigens from stimulating the mother's production of anti-Rh antibodies.

Another feedback reaction is the development of antibodies against the antibodies that form against the original antigen, as follows. Antibodies that are anti-idiotypes (i.e. that are against the antigen receptors on B or T cells) may either suppress or stimulate the immune response, just as a drug which resembles a naturally occurring molecule can either suppress or stimulate the natural target receptor, depending on the drug's specific structure.

Fig. 8-10. The T cytotoxic cell on the target cell's MHC I complex. The cell targeted for death can be a foreign cell, or a host tumor cell with new antigens associated with the tumor cell's MHC I complex. Or the target could be a host cell that has been infected with a virus

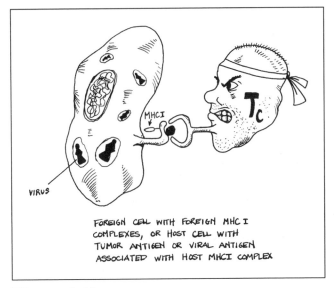

FOREIGN CELL WITH FOREIGN MHC I COMPLEXES, OR HOST CELL WITH TUMOR ANTIGEN OR VIRAL ANTIGEN ASSOCIATED WITH HOST MHCI COMPLEX

Figure 8-10

whose antigen attaches to the MHC I complex. There is a specific T cytotoxic cell for each type of viral antigen. T cytotoxic cells demonstrate a specificity for antigen, just as do the B and Th cell. As is the case for B cells, T cytotoxic cells proliferate to form memory cells with the help of T helper cells. Thus, a T helper cell is first presented with antigen by an antigen-presenting cell, which also stimulates the T helper cell with cytokines (e.g. IL-1). The T helper cell then develops IL-2 receptors on its surface (necessary for response to IL-2) and produces IL-2, which stimulates the production of more T helper cells, which continue to produce IL-2, which stimulates proliferation of the T cytotoxic cells and the expression of the killer quality in T cytotoxic cells. The T-helper cell thus activates B cells, other T helper cells, and T cytotoxic cells. Confusing? See Fig. 8-9.

The various kinds of lymphocytes look alike but can be distinguished by chemical markers on their surfaces. Thus, among other markers, T helper cells contain the "CD4" marker, whereas T suppressor cells and T cytotoxic cells contain the "CD8" marker. Hence the names "T4" and "T8" lymphocytes. Special markers are also useful in distinguishing leukemic cells from normal cells.

Natural killer cell lymphocytes have been mentioned above as being more primitive forms that can kill microorganisms without the specificity of B and T cells. Natural killer cells do not require MHC on the target cells. Natural killer cells do not contain the typical B and T cell markers.

Immune Complexes

Fig. 8-11. The reaction of antibody and antigen can result in large, precipitating complexes or small soluble complexes, depending on the ratio of antibody to antigen. An equal ratio tends to produce a larger, precipitating complex.

Sometimes, all an antibody has to do is to react with an antigen and thereby neutralize it. Often, though, the antibody needs the help of complement or phagocytic cells to properly dispose of the offending antigen. The phagocytic cell engulfs the complex, whereas complement can solubilize complexes and also help attach them to phagocytic cells. Antigen-antibody complexes usually undergo phagocytosis and are removed.

If immune complexes are not removed, they may precipitate and damage normal tissue. Sometimes this results from defective phagocytosis. Damage may also occur through the unrestrained activation of complement by the antigen/antibody complex, and stimulation of neutrophils and macrophages to secrete lysosomal enzymes that damage normal tissue.

Fig. 8-12. Natural and adaptive immune mechanisms do not act independently, but work together. Antibody-antigen complexes interact with complement and with nonspecific cells of natural immunity, such as macrophages, neutrophils, mast cells, or NK cells. For instance:

1) A phagocytic cell (Fig. 8-12) may have:
  a) A **receptor for bacterial antigens,** through which bacteria are directly phagocytosed.
  b) A **receptor for complement**, through which the phagocytic cell deals with a complement-antigen complex, or a complement-antibody-antigen complex. Complement and phagocytic cells, although non-specific actors, are important in the elimination of antigen/antibody complexes.
  c) A **receptor for the Fc portion of antibodies**, through which the phagocytic cell deals with an antibody-antigen complex.
2) Antigen-antibody complexes can activate complement.
3) T cells, being advanced and culturally sophisticated, do not generally interact directly with free-float-

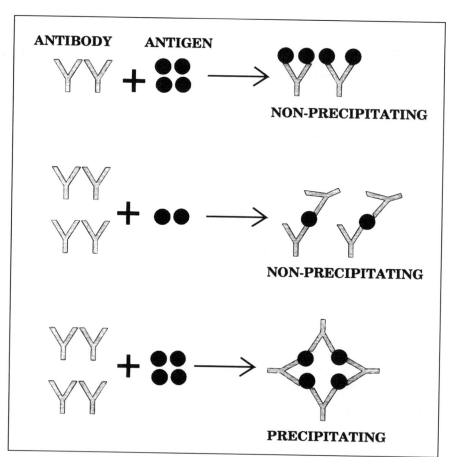

Figure 8-11

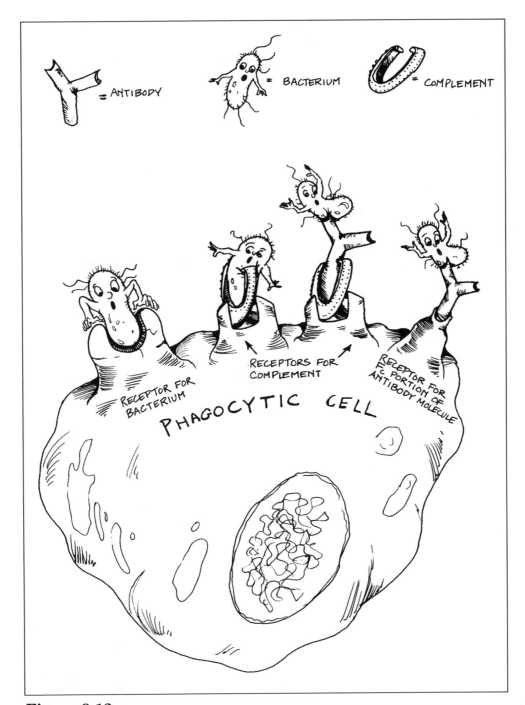

Figure 8-12

ing antigens, but need to be properly introduced to them, commonly via macrophages that carry the antigens to the T cells.

4) Activated B and T cells activate the less specific macrophages and natural killer cells.

In view of the large number of B and T cell variations,

the body cannot maintain a large supply of each one. The ones that exist are strategically located throughout the body, particularly in lymph nodes, which drain the body, and within which there is a meshlike framework that can entrap antigens. When B lymphocytes (situated in lymph node **germinal centers**) are stimulated by specific antigens, those few lymphocytes divide, producing not only antibody-secreting plasma cells, but also memory cells, which persist and can more quickly mount an immune response should the same antigen be presented again.

Lymph node Th cells are mainly located near follicles where they are close to B cells and can exert their helper function. B and T lymphocytes may exit the lymph node via the lymphatic or blood circulations and end up in the general blood circulation, interstitial spaces, other lymph nodes, spleen or other organs. Plasma cells remain mainly in the lymph nodes and spleen, and produce antibody from there.

Lymph nodes, the spleen, and the thymus all have a blood supply, of course. Lymph nodes, though, have afferent and efferent lymphatics, enabling lymph nodes to deal mainly with lymph-borne antigens.

The spleen has no lymphatic circulation and deals mainly with blood-borne antigens. Splenic arterioles end in vascular sinusoids of **red pulp**, which filter blood of nonimmunogenic foreign substances and old red blood cells. Near the red pulp are macrophages, dendritic cells, plasma cells and lymphocytes, in regions termed **white pulp**. Also, the spleen can act as a reservoir for blood.

The thymus has exiting lymphatics but no entering lymphatics.

When Things Go Wrong

A number of factors may interfere with a successful immune response:

1) Microorganisms may adapt.
2) The immune response may be excessive, damaging the host.
3) The immune response may be underactive.

Microorganism Adaptation

Microorganisms may successfully adapt and defend themselves against the host response in the following ways:

a) A bacterial capsule may prevent attachment to host macrophages.

b) The bacterial cell wall may resist digestion and may contain **endotoxins**, toxic lipopolysaccharides found in the cell walls of gram-negative organisms particularly.

c) The bacteria may secrete **exotoxins,** some of which can damage phagocytic cells; others (**ag-**

gressins) alter the environment in a way that promotes spread of the bacteria through the tissues.

d) The microorganism may demonstrate only weak antigenicity.

e) Microorganism antigen variations may thwart the host's reaction just when the host has successfully developed an antibody response to the old antigen.

Excessive host response

The host response may be excessive, damaging the host (even during a normal immune response) with direct toxicity from non-specific components of the natural immunity response. The inflammation and cell lysis caused by excessive complement activation may be harmful. So also may be the toxic effects of excessive cellular and chemical interactions of phagocytic cells with normal tissues.

Complement may be excessively activated in resistant infections or in the continuing stimulation of an autoimmune reaction. Increased complement activity may also occur when feedback inhibitory components of the complement cascade are deficient. In **hereditary angioneurotic edema**, there are attacks of skin and mucosal (e.g. laryngeal) membrane edema from excessive complement activity.

In the **Schwartzman reaction**, there is an overreactive response to microbes; bacterial endotoxin (lipopolysaccharide, LPS) induces the production of tumor necrosis factor (TNF) in phagocytes. TNF in excess causes decreased myocardial contractility, vascular blood coagulation, poor tissue perfusion, and shock ("**endotoxin shock**"). TNF has a selective effect on tumor blood vessels and may be useful in controlling certain tumors, but TNF may also kill the individual through shock.

Damage may also result from hypersensitive components of the acquired immune response:

Damage may be caused by IgE (Type I hypersensitivity reactions), IgG and IgM (Type II hypersensitivity reactions), antibody-antigen complexes (Type III reactions), or by T helper or T cytolytic cells in cell-mediated immunity (Type IV reactions).

Type I reactions (e.g. pollen allergy) are acute reactions **mediated by IgE**. IgE attaches to Fc receptors on the blood basophils and tissue mast cells. When this occurs together with cross-linking of the antigen with the IgE, the mast cell (or basophil) degranulates, releasing vasoactive substances. This can result in a spectrum from rashes to anaphylactic shock, with vasodilatory hypotension and bronchiolar spasm. Nonspecific cells cause the damage, but the condition is initiated by a specific antigen. Type I is the most common form of hypersensitivity. It can flair up within minutes.

Type II reactions (e.g. blood transfusion reactions; autoimmune disease; transplant rejection by antibodies) are **mediated by IgG or IgM**. They may involve reactions against foreign antigens (e.g. **transplant rejection**) or against self-antigens (**autoimmune reactions**). The following are examples:

Autoimmune hemolytic anemia. Autoantibodies to RBC membrane proteins cause hemolysis.

Autoimmune thrombocytopenic purpura. Autoantibodies to platelet surface proteins result in thrombocytopenia.

Diabetes mellitus (insulin resistant). Autoantibodies against insulin receptors may cause diabetes. As it is the receptor that is affected, rather than insulin production, the patient is unresponsive to insulin therapy.

Goodpasture's syndrome. Autoantibodies to collagen in renal glomeruli and lung alveoli result in nephritis and pulmonary hemorrhages.

Grave's disease. Autoantibodies to TSH (thyroid stimulating hormone) receptors on thyroid cells have a **stimulatory** effect on thyroid production, causing hyperthyroidism.

Myasthenia gravis. Autoantibody to neuron acetylcholine receptors causes muscle weakness.

Pemphigus. Autoantibodies to epidermal proteins cause skin and mucous membrane blistering.

Pernicious anemia. Autoantibodies to intrinsic factor deplete intrinsic factor, which is needed for vitamin B_{12} absorption. The symptoms are due to B_{12} deficiency.

Rheumatic fever. This disease is associated with streptococcal pharyngitis. Unlike poststreptococcal glomerulonephritis (see below, as an example of immune complex-mediated disease), rheumatic fever does not involve the kidney, but does cause, among other things, **fever, migratory polyarthritis** and, most seriously, **carditis**. The myocardial inflammation may be due to autoantibodies against myocardial antigens that cross-react with streptococcal antigen, but this is unclear. It is a general problem in such research to determine whether existing autoantibodies actually cause the disease or are the result of tissue damage. (For example, elevated SGPT enzymes, while correlated with liver disease, do not cause the liver disease, but simply are released from liver cells during liver cell damage.)

Excessive production of monoclonal antibodies may be detected as a byproduct of certain lymphoproliferative disorders of plasma cells. In **Waldenstrom's macroglobulinemia**, for instance, there is excess production of monoclonal IgM, coinciding with the anemia and bone marrow infiltration from abnormal, proliferating lymphocytes and plasma cells. The excess IgM may, among other things, cause blood hyperviscosity, resulting in sluggish blood flow, mental confusion, and retinal hemorrhages. **Multiple myeloma** is a plasma cell tumor that invades bone. In addition to hypercalcemia from bone marrow destruction, there is increased production of monoclonal antibody (usually an IgG) and excess production of antibody light chains. The light chains filter through the kidney and are detectable on urine testing (**Bence-Jones protein**). Kidney damage may result from the hypercalcemia and Bence-Jones protein. Rarely, lymphatic malignancies may be associated with the excess production of antibody heavy chains.

Type III reactions (e.g. chronic glomerulonephritis, serum sickness, rheumatoid arthritis, Arthus reaction) are **mediated by antigen/antibody complexes.** Unphagocytosed antigen/antibody complexes may settle in tissues and excessively activate complement. The activated complement in turn activates neutrophils and macrophages to produce tissue-destructive lytic enzymes or phagocytose host cells. Neutrophils and macrophages can also be activated directly by immune complexes without the assistance of complement.

Immune complexes may cause widespread disease, but commonly they particularly affect blood vessels and highly filtering tissues, such as renal glomeruli (urine filtration) and synovial joints (synovial joint fluid). A common picture, therefore, is vasculitis, nephritis, and arthritis.

When the immune complex forms in the blood stream, as in the infusion of foreign serum (**serum sickness**), the pathology may be widespread. On the other hand, the **Arthus reaction** is a localized form of immune complex hypersensitivity. A subcutaneous injection of antigen into an animal with antibody against the antigen results in immune complexes that settle in the tissue vasculature locally, causing vascular inflammation and tissue necrosis.

Examples of Type III reactions include:

Polyarteritis nodosa. An immune complex of hepatitis B surface antigen (HBs Ag) and anti-HBs antibody results in diffuse arteritis.

Post-streptococcal glomerulonephritis. An immune complex of antigens from the streptococcal wall with antibody to them results in glomerulonephritis. Interestingly, the condition does not involve other systemic effects (arteritis, arthritis) and it is believed that rather than the immune complex settling in the glomeruli, the strep antigen may deposit first in the glomeruli and the antibody follows, thereby confining the antigen/antibody complex to the glomeruli.

Rheumatoid arthritis. This condition may involve IgM autoantibodies (called **rheumatoid factors**) to IgG. Although the autoantibodies exist (and assist in the diagnosis of rheumatoid arthritis), it is not clear whether they cause the disease or are a response to tissue damage caused by some other unknown factor(s).

Systemic lupus erythematosis. Autoantibodies to DNA and nucleoproteins result in vasculitis, nephritis, and arthritis, among other things.

Type IV reactions (e.g. graft rejection, contact sensitivity, tuberculin response) are **cell-mediated** reactions. Damage may be caused by cytokines released from T helper cells, by activated T cytolytic cells, or by antibody production that is indirectly stimulated by T cell interaction with B cells.

Cell-mediated hypersensitivity reactions take longer than antibody-mediated reactions, often hours or days, the delay being due to the time required to mobilize cells through the T cell chain of interactions. Contact sensitivity is a variety of this, in which skin Langerhans cells respond to antigen on the skin and initiate a T helper response. An eczematous rash may appear 1–2 days later. Such delayed reactions in skin tests have also been called "**delayed hypersensitivity**."

Tuberculin skin testing is another example of delayed hypersensitivity due to cell-mediated reactions. Tuberculin antigen is injected intradermally, and a classic reaction, in a person who has been exposed to tuberculosis, develops 48-72 hrs later in the form of an indurated reactive area on the skin. The reaction occurs through cell-mediated immunity.

In the clinical disease **tuberculosis**, cell-mediated immunity attempts to eliminate the tubercle bacillus by activating macrophages, which ingest the bacilli. If the ingested bacilli remain alive, the body may attempt a chronic inflammatory response, walling off the affected cells in damaging granulomas (Fig. 8-6), in the lung and elsewhere. **Sarcoidosis** (nodules in lung, eyes, skin), **Crohn's disease** and **ulcerative colitis** (bowel), and **temporal arteritis** (arteries) are other examples of granulomatous diseases that are believed to involve cell-mediated immunity.

Nongranulomatous diseases that may have an origin in cell-mediated immune responses include multiple sclerosis, myasthenia gravis, Grave's disease, and viral myocarditis. Note that myasthenia gravis and Grave's disease were also mentioned under type II (IgG) reactions, and there is some ambiguity here in classification, since T helper cells can stimulate B cells to produce autoantibody.

Autoimmunity

Autoimmunity may be caused by either B or T cells, or both. Potential mechanisms include the following:

1) The autoimmunity may not be against self antigens. Rather, a foreign antigen, e.g. virus or drug, attaches to the host cell. The immune response is against the foreign antigen, and in the process kills the host cell, too.
2) The foreign antigen may resemble a host antigen in some respect, and the immune response thus includes the host as well.
3) Certain antigens (e.g. bacterial lipopolysaccharide) can induce a generalized clonal proliferation of B cells (**polyclonal activation**), including the small population of self-reacting B cells that otherwise would be insufficient in number to mount an autoimmune response.
4) Antigens that appear later in development or are sequestered in the body and never participated in fetal self-tolerance may later generate an autoimmune reaction. For example, in severe ocular injury in which there is laceration of the choroid layer of the eye with permanent loss of vision, ophthalmologists may sometimes opt to remove the damaged eye, because leaving it in may lead to an autoimmune reaction against the opposite eye (post-traumatic uveitis) from antigens originally sequestered in the choroid but now released.
5) Factors that suppress the immune response (e.g. T suppressor cells) may be deficient.

Immunodeficiency

Defects in the immune system may occur at any point in the immune mechanism—at the nonspecific level of complement, granulocytes and macrophages, or at the specific level of B and T lymphocytes. Immune deficiency renders the patient susceptible to infections and, in some cases, tumors. The specific infection that develops may depend on which component of the immune system is defective. In some disorders, the immune system is not the only system affected, and diseases may develop with components other than infection and tumors.

Deficiency in phagocytic cells and complement will cause susceptibility to bacterial infections, since phagocytic cells and complement are the first-line defense against bacteria. Moreover, since complement is also important in the removal of immune complexes, patients with complement deficits may also develop diseases of immune complex deposition, with vasculitis, nephritis, and arthritis.

If the defect lies in one of the **inhibitors** of a step in the complement cascade, there may be excessive accumulation of the complement component acting at that step. Examples include **hereditary angioneurotic edema** (acute episodes of edema in the skin and mucosa), and **paroxysmal nocturnal hemoglobinuria** (hemolysis with appearance of hemoglobin in the urine).

Hereditary defects in phagocytic cells include **leukocyte adhesion deficiency**, in which defective leukocyte function results in increased susceptibility to infection. **Chediak-Higashi Syndrome** is a hereditary disorder of lysosomes that affects neutrophils, monocytes, lymphocytes, and other kinds of cells, resulting not only in infections, but hemorrhage (platelet involvement), neurologic impairment, and albinism.

Individuals with T cell deficiencies are open to many infections but still may be able to handle microbes with polysaccharides as primary antigens, because the defense against polysaccharide antigens involves antibody that is T cell-independent. Defects in (B cell) humoral immunity render the patient more susceptible to pyogenic **bacterial** infections, or organisms for which B cells and their associated antibodies are the main defense. Defects in (T cell) cell-mediated immunity are more associated with defective responses to **viruses** (and viral-induced tumors), and organisms for which T cells are important in the defense, including intracellular bacteria (such as Tb), fungi, and protozoa. It must be remembered, though, that T cells are also important in B cell activation, and, therefore, T cells deficiencies can result in defects in humoral immunity.

AIDS

Defects in B or T cells can be secondary to chemotherapy, irradiation, malnutrition, hereditary factors, or invasive cancer. In the case of **AIDS (Acquired ImmunoDeficiency Syndrome)**, T helper cells are destroyed or impaired by the AIDS virus (presently called the **HIV**, or **Human Immunodeficiency Virus**), which enters the T helper cell (also referred to as the CD4+ T cell, or T4 cell) via the cell's CD4 surface receptor.

Antibodies first appear against the HIV virus about 3–20 weeks after exposure to the virus, which is trans-

mitted through the exchange of body fluids (e.g. semen, through sexual contact; blood, through shared intravenous needles; breast milk or in utero transmission from an AIDS-carrying mother).

The first manifestation of HIV infections may be a flu-like illness, or the patient may be asymptomatic. A latent phase may then exist for up to 10 years or longer. Many patients in this time interval develop lymphadenopathy. Some may also develop **ARC (AIDS-Related Complex)**, consisting of fever, weight loss, and diarrhea; and the number of T4 cells decrease. Eventually, most patients develop full-blown AIDS with profound loss of T4 cells.

The patient with AIDS becomes susceptible to a variety of infections, some of which are otherwise rarely seen, such as the protozoan, **Pneumocystis pneumoniae**, a very common cause of death in AIDS. Other unusual protozoal infections (Toxoplasma, Cryptosporidium), bacterial infections (Tb, Salmonella, Nocardia), fungal infections (Candida, Cryptococcus, Coccidioides, Histoplasma), viral infections (Cytomegalovirus, Herpes simplex, Varicella), and helminth infections (Strongyloides) are also common. The patient may also develop **Kaposi's sarcoma**, a rarely seen tumor.

The ratio of T4 (T-helper) to T8 (T-cytotoxic and T-suppressor) cells is important in the diagnosis of AIDS, since T4 (helper) lymphocytes are destroyed by the virus. Normally a person has about a 2/1 ratio of T4 to T8 cells. This ratio may decrease to as much as 0.5 in patients with AIDS.

B and T cell defects can also be hereditary. In the case of hereditary B cell deficiency, there may be a diffuse hypogammaglobulinemia; or the defect may be more selective, involving IgG, IgA, or IgM.

An example of a hereditary T cell deficit is the **DeGeorge syndrome**, in which there is failure of thymic development, and hence a deficiency in T cells. Patients with this condition, in addition to various congenital anomalies, also have impaired cell-mediated immunity, with normal or abnormal immunoglobulin levels.

In other hereditary conditions, there may be a combined deficiency of both B and T cells. In some of them, there may be multiple other problems. For instance, in the **Wiskott-Aldrich syndrome**, there are B and T cell defects, but also thrombocytopenia. In **ataxia telangiectasia**, there are, in addition to B and T cell defects, vascular malformations (hemangiomas) and neurologic problems.

IMMUNE TESTS

The fact that antibodies combine with antigens has suggested numerous laboratory methods that test either for specific antibody or specific antigen in the patient, including **precipitation, agglutination, and neutralization tests**, and the use of fluorescent, radioactive, or enzymatic labels:

1) **Precipitation tests.** Some tests detect a specific antibody (or antigen) in the patient's serum by precipitating it in the lab with corresponding antigen (or antibody) either in a test tube or in agar diffusion. In agar diffusion, separate diffusing sources of antigen and antibody precipitate where their diffusing fronts meet each other in equal concentrations (as precipitation is greatest when the concentration of antigen and antibody are equal—see Fig. 8-11). For example, **alpha fetal protein (AFP)** is elevated in the serum of women pregnant with fetuses that have neural tube defects, such as spina bifida. It may be detected through precipitation by diffusing it against anti-AFP antibody.

Precipitation tests may be facilitated by first separating the proteins in the patient's serum by **electrophoresis**. The separated components of electrophoresed field are then used in the precipitation tests.

The electrophoresis in itself may provide useful information about antibodies. Most immunoglobulins fall in the gamma globulin zone. A sharp spike in the gamma globulin area on elecrophoresis suggests the overproduction of a single antibody, as might occur in a tumor of a single clone of plasma cells. A broad increase is more consistent with a general (polyclonal) response of antibody production.

Immunonephelometry (IN) is a technique that quantitates the amount of antigen-antibody complex in solution through measuring the light-scattering characteristics of the complexes.

2) **Agglutination tests.** Because not all antibody-antigen complexes precipitate readily, a visible reaction may be obtained if the antibody (or antigen) is attached to something that will **agglutinate** (clump) when the antibody-antigen reaction occurs (e.g. red blood cells, bacteria, or antigen-coated beads). **Flocculation** is a variation of agglutination, in which the aggregate is visible but smaller, in suspended fluffy, or colloid, form. Examples:

a) **Testing for A and B RBC antigens in blood typing.** One observes whether agglutination occurs when mixing the patient's RBCs with known anti-A or anti-B antisera.

b) **Testing for C-reactive protein (CRP).** CRP rises in the acute phase of inflammation (also in certain malignancies). It can be detected by first binding anti-CRP antibodies to latex particles. The particles will agglutinate on exposure to a patient's serum that has C-reactive protein. A positive test helps confirm the impression of an inflammation. Conversion to a negative test helps confirm the remission of the condition.

c) **Heterophil antibody test** for mononucleosis. Heterophil antibodies, which occur in mononucleosis, are antibodies that react with a number of diverse antigens. Agglutination of sheep RBCs by the patient's serum suggests the presence of heterophil antibodies and mononucleosis. The **mono spot test** is a more rapid-acting variation of this test that uses horse RBCs.

d) **Syphilis tests.** In the **VDRL** screening test, cardiolipin, an antigen released from the treponema organism, is added to samples of the patient's serum. If microflocculation appears, the test suggests syphilis but is not highly specific. False positives can occur with a number of other kinds of disease processes, including viral illnesses and autoimmune diseases. Also, false negatives can occur early in the course of syphilis. The **RPR** test is similar to the VDRL, but involves a macroscopically visible reaction using a card kit, whereas the VDRL requires glass slides and a microscope. The **FTA-ABS** (fluorescent treponemal antibody absorption) and **TPI** (treponema pallidum immobilization) tests are more specific for syphilis, since they use actual treponema-specific antigens. In the FTA-ABS, the patient's serum is put on a slide with dried T. pallidum. If antibody is present, it sticks to the treponema and is detected by adding to the slide fluorescent-labeled antihuman gamma-globulin. The TPI tests for antibodies to syphilis in the patient's serum through the immobilization of living motile treponema by a mixture of the patient's serum and complement.

e) The **latex agglutination (latex fixation) test** for rheumatoid factor in rheumatoid arthritis. Rheumatoid factor is an IgM that is anti-IgG. IgG is bound in the test to tiny latex particles, which agglutinate on adding patient's serum that contains rheumatoid factor.

f) Test for **anti-nuclear antibodies (ANA)** in lupus erythematosis. Latex particles are coated with deoxyribonucleoprotein. The test is positive for ANA if agglutination occurs on adding the patient's serum. A negative reaction suggests that lupus is not present, but a positive reaction can occur in other conditions, including rheumatoid arthritis. The **LE prep** test detects anti-nuclear antibody by the characteristic histologic appearance of neutrophils that have phagocytosed ANA/nucleoprotein complexes.

g) **HCG (human chorionic gonadotropin) hormone assay for pregnancy.** This popular test for pregnancy is a variation on the standard agglutination tests, and involves **agglutination inhibition**. It tests for HCG, which is present during pregnancy. Latex particles are first coated with HCG. The patient's urine is mixed with anti-HCG. If the urine contains HCG, it neutralizes the anti-HCG and, when added to the latex particles, will not agglutinate them. Thus the **absence** of agglutination during the test constitutes a positive test for pregnancy.

h) **Widal test.** This test detects antibodies to salmonella when agglutination of Salmonella typhosa occurs on the latter's exposure to the patient's serum. Similar tests are used for detection of brucellosis and tularemia antibodies.

i) **Weil-Felix test.** This is a test for rickettsial disease. Dilutions of the patient's serum are exposed to Proteus OX-19, a bacterium that has antigen in common to rickettsiae. Agglutination is consistent with rickettsial disease (but also with Proteus).

j) **Cold agglutinin test.** This tests for **antibodies to Mycoplasma pneumoniae** in the patient's serum, by noting their special property of reversibly agglutinating red blood cells when the patient's serum and RBCs are exposed to cold.

3) The suspected antibody (or antigen) may be detected by noting the **neutralization** of the activity of one of the ingredients of the antigen-antibody reaction. Examples:

a) **Antistreptolysin O titer.** Streptolysin O, a product of streptococci, lyses red blood cells. Antistreptolysin O antibodies (ASO) develop during streptococcal infections. ASO in the patient's blood can be detected by mixing the patient's serum with streptolysin O and human red blood cells and noting that hemolysis will be **inhibited** by the patient's serum. It is the streptolysin O that is neutralized in the test.

b) **Diagnostic tests for specific viruses, through identification of their antibodies.** For instance, the influenza virus contains hemagglutinin (HA), which can agglutinate RBCs. The **HA inhibition test** examines for the presence of anti-HA in the patient's serum. The patient's serum is mixed with viruses containing HA. If anti-HA is present, it neutralizes the HA and significant hemagglutination will not occur when RBCs are added. It is the virus that is neutralized in the test.

c) Tests for **antibodies against coagulation factors** as a cause of coagulation disorders. A patient with a suspected antibody against a coagulation factor can be tested by exposing normal plasma to the patient's serum, in which case clotting will be inhibited by the inhibiting antibody in the patient's serum. In this case, it is the coagulation factor that is neutralized.

d) Tests for **antibodies against sperm**, as a cause of fertility problems. Male or female sera are tested for anti-sperm antibodies by examining for sperm immobilization when donor sperm is mixed with the serum samples. It is the sperm that is neutralized in the test.

e) **Complement fixation tests** are useful in the **detection of a wide variety of viral antibodies.** The idea is that hemolysin antibody causes lysis of red blood cells provided that complement is also present. This lysis can be inhibited in the presence of immune complexes, which combine with complement and thereby prevent complement from facilitating the lysis. In the test, sheep RBCs are coated with hemolysin and mixed with guinea pig complement, the patient's serum, and the viral antigen of interest. If the patient's serum contains antibody to the viral antigen, it will combine with the viral antigen, form an immune complex which will neutralize ("fix") the complement, and thereby inhibit the hemolysis.

A related kind of test can be used to assess the **amount of complement activity in a patient's serum**. One notes the ability of the patient's serum to induce lysis in hemolysin-coated RBCs.

4) The laboratory antibody (antigen) that is added to the patient's serum or tissue to test for the presence of corresponding antigen (or antibody) may first be **labeled** with something that will be easily detectable (e.g. fluorescein, radioactive markers, enzymes that can be detected by their particular chemical reactions).

For example, in the **double-antibody sandwich ELISA** (Enzyme-Linked Immunosorbent Assay) test, one coats the wall of a polystyrene microplate well with a specific **antibody**, say antibody to hepatitis B antigen (anti-HBsAg) if one is examining a patient's serum for HBsAg. The patient's serum is then applied to the well. If the serum contains HBsAg, it will stick to the coated antibody. The HbsAg can then be detected by applying to the well a second antibody, an anti-HBsAg that is labeled with enzyme. If HBsAg is present, the enzyme-labeled anti-HBsAg will not wash out and can be detected through testing for enzyme activity.

In the **indirect ELISA** test, the microplate well is instead coated with a known **antigen** (HBsAg, if one is testing for anti-HBsAg antibody), and the patient's serum is then added. Following that, enzyme-labeled anti-human globulin is applied. If the anti-human globulin sticks, as assessed by the presence of enzyme activity, then the test is positive for anti-HBsAg antibody in the patient's serum.

In the **Western blotting technique**, an elecrophoresed sample is picked up ("blotted") from its electrophoretic gel onto a membrane that now becomes a duplicate of the electrophoretic pattern. Specific labeled antibody is then applied to the membrane to test for the presence of specific corresponding antigen. The separation of the antigen from the gel allows the antigen to react better.

In testing for antigen or antibody, it is often useful to compare a patient's serum sample with known standards. It may also help to compare the patient's serum sample in the acute phase of an illness with a later phase, because changes in antibody or antigen titers can provide a better idea of the course of the disease, and whether or not existing antibodies are due to an old illness. Testing serial dilutions of the patient's serum is also useful, becaue the diagnosis often is more firmly established if reaction still occurs beyond a certain degree of dilution.

Immunosuppression and Immunostimulation

Immunosuppression is an important therapeutic modality that is used to diminish the harmful effects of immune hypersensitivity.

Disadvantages of immunosuppression include rendering the host susceptible to infection by damaging the immune system:

Approaches to immunosuppressive treatment include:

1) Deplete the lymphocyte population in general (antilymphocyte serum, antimitotic agents, irradiation, thoracic duct drainage).
2) Remove antibodies in general from plasma by plasma exchange.
3) Interfere with the function of phagocytes in general by administering corticosteroids.
4) Interfere with the activities of lymphocytes. For example, cyclosporin A appears to interfere with T helper production of cytokines as well as with presentation of antigen to the T helper cell.
5) Generally suppress the immune response by injection of T suppressor cells.
6) Specifically suppress the immune response to the particular antigen in the graft by:
   a) Administering specific antibody to block antigenic sites on the graft or to block specific receptor idiotypes on B and T cells.
   b) Administering specific antigen that is coupled to cytotoxic agents to destroy specific lymphocytes.
7) Induce tolerance to an immune response by administering massive doses of an antigen or small dosages given repeatedly. Clinical **desensitization** is an approach designed to decrease IgE levels in allergy by administering increasing quantities of the offending antigen in subcutaneous injections over a course of several weeks or months. The exact mechanism of action is not known, but it is known that the exact dose of antigen and how it is given may determine whether the response is stimulatory or suppressive to the immune system.

Sometimes a patient may become **anergic** (immunologically unresponsive) to an overwhelming infection. For example, in diffuse overwhelming tuberculosis, the patient may no longer exhibit a response to a tuberculin test.

Improvement in the function of the immune system is possible through various **immunostimulation** methods:

1) **Passive immunization** through administration of antibody (e.g. tetanus, snakebite, hepatitis B antiserum) is useful to combat an **existing** infection.
2) **Active immunization** (vaccination) is useful to **prevent** future infection. Attenuated or killed microorganisms, or antigenic components of the microorganism are injected, thereby strengthening the immune system's future response should it encounter the live virulent strain.
3) Introduction of cells found in the immune response, e.g. grafting of bone marrow or thymus.
4) The use of **adjuvants**, which are substances that enhance the antigenic response. Adjuvants may include substances not normally part of the normal immune response (e.g. oil emulsions, liposomes, as well as cytokines).

Transfusion and Blood Grouping

There are many blood group antigens but ABO and Rh factors are the most commonly involved in transfusion reactions.

A-B-O Factors:

A and/or B antigens occur on RBCs. If you **don't** have these antigens (type O blood), then you **do** have antibodies to them in your blood in a similar way as you would have antibodies to other foreign antigens that are "non-self." The appearance of significant quantities of antibodies may relate to exposure to small quantities of the antigens in the diet, for instance, during postnatal life.

A and B antiGENS are called "agglutinoGENS." The corresponding antibodies are called "agglutinins." Individuals with type A, B, or AB blood contain red blood cells with A, B, or both A and B antigens respectively. Their blood will agglutinate if transfused into a type O individual, who has agglutinins to both A and B antigens. Type O individuals are "**universal donors**" since their red cells contain neither A nor B antigens and will not agglutinate when transfused.

Rh Factor:

The ABO type of incompatibility factors occur naturally. The Rh agglutinins do not, requiring significant exposure to Rh antigens, generally by direct blood transfusion, before enough antibody can form. Hence, with the first pregnancy, Rh incompatibility is not a problem.

People with the Rh antigen are called Rh positive (Rh+). The main Rh antigen is called Type D antigen. There are other less potent ones. The term Rh+ generally refers to the presence of the Type D antigen. An Rh+ mother won't develop Rh antibodies, so her fetus will be unaffected, regardless of whether it is Rh+ or Rh-. If the mother is Rh-, then in response to the fetal cells of an Rh+ fetus, she will produce Rh antibodies. Her antibody production will not occur in time to affect the first fetus but can affect the second pregnancy with an Rh+ fetus, since the antibodies are present for the second pregnancy. If the fetus is affected, this is **erythroblastosis fetalis,** a hemolytic condition of red blood cells. The term "erthroblastosis" refers to the nucleated RBC precursors in the blood that the infant develops to replace the RBCs damaged by the maternal antibodies. **Kernicterus** (damaging deposition of bilirubin in the brain, particularly in the basal ganglia) may arise from the jaundice that appears from the RBC breakdown. Even though the affected baby is Rh+, transfuse the baby with Rh-blood, because if you use Rh+ blood, it might react with Rh+ antibodies still circulating from the mother.

A transfusion of Rh+ blood into an Rh− person (who has never contacted Rh+ blood before) causes no significant immediate reaction since it takes months for the antibody to develop to a significant degree. Within months, though, there may be a reaction. Renal shutdown can occur from a transfusion reaction due to plugging of renal tubules with hemoglobin, in addition to renal vasoconstriction and circulatory shock that may arise from toxic products of the RBC breakdown.

Transplantation

Just as one can type RBC groups, one can tissue-type organs, examining for similarities in the HLA (Human Leukocyte Antigen; MHC) group of antigens, which are the most important antigens for tissue typing. The testing makes convenient use of lymphocytes, which contain the HLA antigens. If the patient's lymphocytes lyse when presented with a mixture of complement and antiserum against a specific HLA antigen, this suggests that the specific HLA antigen is present. HLA typing is thus useful to help maximize effectiveness in matching tissue donors and recipients. It is also used to help resolve paternity disputes. Specific HLA types are also useful in predicting the likelihood of developing certain diseases, such as ankylosing spondylitis, which are associated with particular HLA molecules.

CHAPTER 9.   NEUROPHYSIOLOGY

Fig. 9-1. The neuron, the basic unit of transfer of information in the nervous system. Electrophysiologic impulses (action potentials) travel down a neuron from its dendrites to the cell body and axon. Information then is chemically transmitted to other neurons via connections called **synapses**.

An axon's action potential travels in an "all-or-none manner". That is, a stimulus either is too weak to generate an action potential, or it generates one, in which case the impulse travels with a fixed amplitude, regardless of the strength of the stimulus. The strength of a stimulus is instead encoded in the **frequency** of discharge; the stronger the stimulus, the greater the frequency of action potentials.

See Fig. 5-5 for a review of the major events in the generation of an action potential.

Fig. 9-2. Saltatory conduction in myelinated nerve fibers. In unmyelinated fibers, the axon potential spreads smoothly along the course of the axon. In myelinated fibers, the action potential cannot flow along segments of the nerve that contain myelin layers, which are produced by Schwann cells that wrap around the axon in an insulatory fashion. Instead, the action potential jumps across the myelin segments to nodes of Ranvier, which are the areas between the Schwann cells. This hopping along of the action potential (**saltatory conduction**) is much faster than non-myelinated conduction.

When an action potential reaches the next synapse, it causes the release of a neurochemical transmitter which act on the next cell in the chain to alter its membrane potential, which in turn must be reduced to a threshold level to fire. A single action potential is not enough to do the job. Many action potentials must act near-simultaneously. This may be accomplished through the near-simultaneous firing of many synapses on a single cell (**spatial summation**), or through the rapid succession of action potentials coming through relatively few synapses (**temporal summation**). Excitatory spatial and temporal summations are said to **facilitate** the firing of the target neuron.

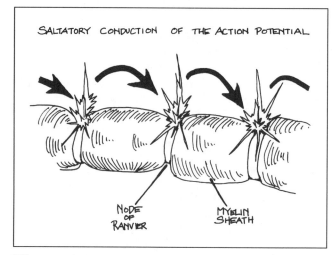

Figure 9-2

Now you can see the logic of coding the strength of a stimulus through frequency of action potentials. The greater the frequency of action potentials, the greater will be their summating facilitatory influence on the firing at the next synapse. Such summated excitatory changes in the postsynaptic neuron's membrane potential are the membrane's **EPSP (excitatory post-synaptic potential)**. The EPSP must be balanced against inhibitory impulses on the same neuron that arise from other synapses and tend to increase the negativity of the postsynaptic neuron's membrane potential. This inhibitory effect is the **IPSP (inhibitory post-synaptic potential)**. The net sum of EPSPs and IPSPs, arising from numerous inputs (a single neuron may have as many as 100,000 synaptic inputs) determines if the cell will fire.

Fig. 9-3. The central nervous system (CNS). The CNS includes the cerebrum, cerebellum, brain stem, and spinal cord plus a few scary-sounding structure situated between the brain stem and cerebrum, namely, the diencephalon (which includes everything with the name "thalamus;" i.e.the thalamus, hypothalamus, epithalamus and subthalamus) and the basal ganglia (which includes the caudate nucleus, the globus pallidus, the putamen, claustrum, and amygdala).

Neurotransmitters

Acetylcholine, **norepinephrine**, and **glutamate** are widespread, mainly excitatory neurotransmitters. Predominantly inhibitory neurotransmitters include **dopamine** (produced in midbrain substantia nigra

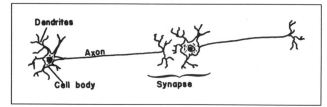

Figure 9-1

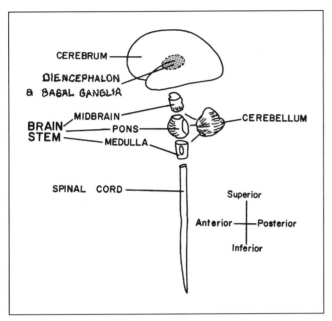

Figure 9-3

cells, which project to the caudate nucleus and putamen areas of the basal ganglia), gamma-aminobutyric acid (**GABA**, widespread), **glycine** (in spinal cord) and **serotonin** (in cells of the median raphe of the brain stem which project to the hypothalamus and other areas).

The **locus ceruleus**, which is situated in the pons, is one the the two pigmented areas of the brain (the other is the substantia nigra in the midbrain). The locus ceruleus is a norepinephrine-producing nucleus that sends widespread excitatory projections to many brain areas, but inhibitory projections to others, and may be important in facilitating wakefulness and attention, as well as the active (REM) phase of sleep. It has been called the adrenal gland of the brain.

Deficiency of dopamine occurs in **Parkinson's disease**, where there is degeneration of the pigmented cells of the substantia nigra of the midbrain.

Decreases in serotonin and norepinephrine may be associated with depression. Thus, the leading antidepressant medications have serotonin and/or norepinephrine-like effects. For instance, desipramine (Norpramin) has norepinephrine-like effects. Fluoxetine (Prozac) has serotonin-like effects. Monoamine oxidase is a naturally-occurring enzyme that metabolizes serotonin and norepinephrine. MAO inhibitors are drugs that block this enzyme and thus have both serotonin-like and norepinephrine-like effects. Endorphins and enkephalins are produced in the hypothalamus and other areas of the brain. They have opioid-like effects of analgesia and sedation.

Neuronal Circuitry Patterns

Axons commonly pass through many synaptic stations on the way from one point to another. These stations are not mere relay points but are important integrative areas, where negative feedback and other modifying influences act on the traveling train of information.

Negative feedback is an important aspect of the organization of neural circuitry and is an important concept in body homeostasis in general. In biochemical reactions, for instance, the end product of a reaction chain frequently feeds back to inhibit earlier components of the chain, thereby insuring that the reaction does not get out of control. Similarly, in the neuronal circuitry, impulses along a particular path frequently feedback to inhibit the firing along the same path, thereby keeping the firing within narrow physiologic limits.

Fig. 9-4. A neuron may synapse on another neuron's dendrites, cell body, or synaptic ending.

Fig. 9-5. The integrative patterns of neuronal circuitry, which lie between the sensory input and motor output may consists of many kinds of patterns ("+" = excitatory synapse; "−" = inhibitory synapse): A. **Negative feedback** sets limits on the activity of neural impulses. B. **Lateral inhibition** of nearby pathways prevents neural impulses from spreading laterally and thereby keeps the information focused along a relatively narrow path. This is important, for instance, in allowing one to finely discriminate touch between two points on the skin that are close to one another. It also enables one to discriminate fine pinpoints of light and contours that are flashed on the retina, and to discern contrast. C. Pathway **convergence.** Multiple inputs can thus influence the activity of a single cell. D. Pathway **divergence.** A single small neural discharge can thus influence a wide area (e.g. the **reticular activating**

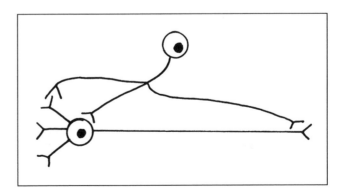

Figure 9-4

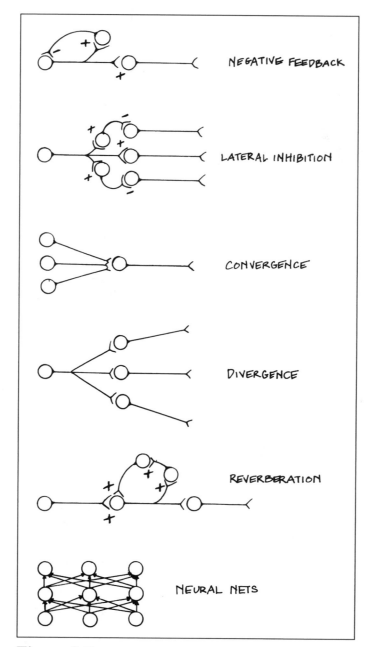

Figure 9-5

system is a neuronal pathway that originates in the brain stem and spreads to influence wide areas of the brain.) E. **Reverberatory circuits** help to sustain a continuing discharge along a neural pathway. Relatively prolonged discharge can also occur through increased numbers of synapses in a pathway, as each synapse entails a certain delay in the passage of information.

Fig. 9-6. Cone sensitivities in the retina. The visual system provides an excellent example of more complex levels of organization of neural pathway connections. The human visual system can perceive hundreds of gradations of colors of the spectrum. Yet it accomplishes this with only 3 kinds of cone photoreceptors in the retina, termed "red", "green", and "blue" photoreceptors. Each receptor type is most sensitive to stimulation at a specific wavelength of light. E.g. light of 650nm wavelength, in the red spectrum, will stimulate red cones. Light at 550 nm, corresponding to yellow, will stimulate both red and green cones. Light at 490nm in the green

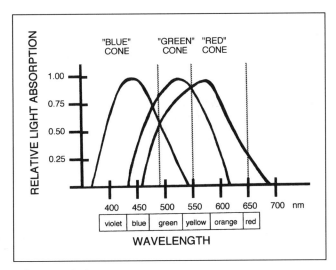

Figure 9-6

range, will stimulate all three cone types to different degrees, but mainly stimulate the green cone receptors. The degree of stimulation of each of the three cone types determines the strength of the neuronal impulses along that cone's connections with the nervous system. The key point is that the ability to distinguish hundreds of different colors does not require the presence of hundreds of different kinds of receptors. Each color is coded as a ratio of the relative strengths of the impulses arising from each of three types of cones. Each different ratio translates into a different pattern of impulses in the brain, which translates into a unique kind of conscious color perception. The color white does not correspond to any known wavelength, but is the result of the stimulation of all three cone types to an equal degree by a mixture of all colors of the spectrum, or alternatively, by a mixture of three different wavelengths that correspond to the peaks of sensitivity of the three cone types.

Visual information is integrated in the visual cortex in ever more complex ways. "Simple" cells in the primary visual cortex may respond, for instance, only to a vertical line of light shined on a particular area of the retina. At steps beyond the simple cell, there are "complex" cells that may respond, for instance, only to a vertical line that is moving in a particular direction. More complex shapes may be recognized by "hypercomplex" cells. There is some humerous speculation (remembering that there often is many a truth hidden in a jest) that there may be a "grandmother" cell that responds only to the sight of a grandmother. Certainly, visual integration becomes quite complex as one moves beyond the visual cortex, toward the **angular gyrus** of the cerebrum (Fig. 9-24). Lesions there, while not interfer-

ing with a patient's ability to read a Snellen chart with 20/20 visual acuity, may interfere with the patient's ability to understand the written word.

Sensory Receptors

Sensory receptors are specialized sensory nerve endings that generate electrophysiologic nerve impulses from various forms of incoming stimuli:

1) Mechanical stimuli (touch, vibration, and pressure receptors in the skin, joints and other areas; carotid and aortic baroreceptors that respond to blood pressure changes; stretch receptors in muscle; sound wave receptors in the cochlea of the inner ear; receptors for movement and gravitational effects in the vestibular apparatus of the inner ear).
2) Thermal stimuli (hot and cold receptors in the skin).
3) Chemical stimuli (taste buds in tongue; olfactory receptors in the nose; oxygen receptors in the carotid body; pH receptors in the brain stem; osmolality receptors in hypothalamus).
4) Electromagnetic stimuli (photoreceptors in the retina).

Fig. 9-7. Schematic view of receptors and motor fibers in the control of muscle movement. In order to achieve smooth, precise control of muscle action, it is insufficient simply to have motor nerves innervating skeletal muscle fibers. Motion would be too jerky. It is important to have continuous feedback during muscle contraction as to the **degree of muscle stretch**, the **speed of stretching**, and the **degree of muscle tension**. The degree of stretch is not the same as the degree of tension. For instance, if both the biceps and its antagonist, the triceps muscle, contract simultaneously, the biceps muscle may not change its degree of stretch, but its tension will increase.

The **Golgi tendon organs** (Fig. 9-8) are **tension** detectors in muscle tendons. **Muscle spindles** (Fig. 9-7) are **stretch** detectors within the bulk of the muscle.

Each muscle spindle contains two sorts of sensory receptors—**primary** and **secondary nerve endings** (Fig. 9-7). Both the primary (type Ia; annulospiral) and secondary (type II) nerve endings relay information about the degree of muscle stretching. The primary nerve endings also relay information about the **rate** of muscle stretching. Thus, if the muscle is stretched significantly but is just resting in the static stretched state, both the primary and secondary receptors detect this and relay to the spinal cord, cerebellum, and other centers, negative feedback information that will result in resistance to the amount of stretch, by increasing

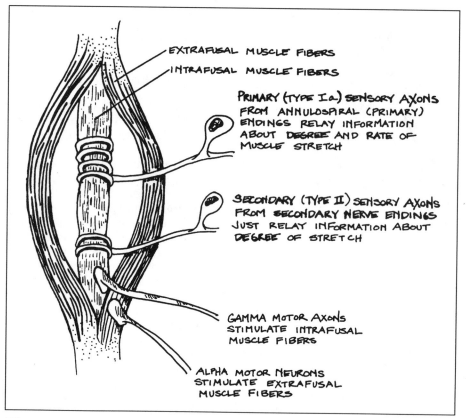

EXTRAFUSAL MUSCLE FIBERS

INTRAFUSAL MUSCLE FIBERS

PRIMARY (TYPE Ia) SENSORY AXONS FROM ANNULOSPIRAL (PRIMARY) ENDINGS RELAY INFORMATION ABOUT DEGREE AND RATE OF MUSCLE STRETCH

SECONDARY (TYPE II) SENSORY AXONS FROM SECONDARY NERVE ENDINGS JUST RELAY INFORMATION ABOUT DEGREE OF STRETCH

GAMMA MOTOR AXONS STIMULATE INTRAFUSAL MUSCLE FIBERS

ALPHA MOTOR NEURONS STIMULATE EXTRAFUSAL MUSCLE FIBERS

Figure 9-7

the muscle contraction. If the muscle is **suddenly** stretched significantly, i.e. the rate of stretch is significant, there is an additional strong input from the primary receptors to resist this. The **knee jerk reflex** is an example: On tapping the patellar tendon, this stretches the quadriceps muscle, and the primary nerve endings in the muscle spindles respond, relaying information that results in a sudden knee jerk contraction of the quadriceps. A similar reflex can be obtained by tapping the muscle directly.

The muscle spindle contains a modified grouping of small muscle fibers, called **intrafusal fibers**, as opposed to the regular **extrafusal fibers** of the main skeletal muscle bulk. The primary and secondary nerve endings wrap around the intrafusal fibers, responding to changes in their length. Stretching of the extrafusal fibers stretches the intrafusal fibers and stimulates the primary and secondary nerve endings. **Alpha motor fibers** innervate the extrafusal muscle fibers. **Gamma motor fibers** innervate the intrafusal fibers.

Generally, gamma motor fibers fire whenever alpha motor fibers fire. This ensures that the length of the in-

trafusal fibers keeps pace with changes in the length of extrafusal fibers so that the intrafusal fibers don't get either too floppy or too tight.

As a general rule, when an individual tries to flex or extend a joint, inhibitory impulses are relayed to the antagonistic muscle (unless one tries purposefully to contract both the flexor and extensor muscles at the same time). Thus, on attempted biceps flexion (or for that matter the reflex in which the biceps tendon is tapped), the biceps muscle contracts, whereas the triceps, its antagonist, is inhibited. This rule is useful in unmasking malingering. For instance, if a patient claims paralysis of biceps flexion, then, in true weakness, both the biceps and triceps muscles will be felt to be flaccid on attempted biceps flexion. However, if the patient is malingering, one may note that the patient is "trying hard" to flex the elbow, and indeed the elbow joint does not flex on attempted flexion, but this is due to simultaneous vigorous contraction of both the biceps and triceps, which cannot happen physiologically either in biceps weakness or on normal biceps flexion. This nonphysiologic pattern may be seen on TV "professional" wrestling shows.

Fig. 9-8. The Golgi tendon organ. Whereas the muscle spindle reacts against **stretching** by decreasing extrafusal muscle **stretch** (through extrafusal muscle contraction), the Golgi tendon organ reacts against increased muscle **tension** by decreasing the extrafusal muscle **tension**, two homeostatic negative feedback mechanisms. In a sense, though, the muscle spindle and Golgi tendon organ have opposite effects, since muscle spindle stimulation decreases stretch, whereas the way the Golgi apparatus decreases muscle tension is by allowing the muscle to stretch. Together the muscle spindle and Golgi tendon organ contribute to the smooth, continuous feedback regulation of muscle movement.

Information about position and movement of the joints comes not only from Golgi tendon organs and muscle spindles, but also from specialized receptors in and around the joint capsules and ligaments. This information enters the spinal cord and goes to both the cerebellum (unconscious perception) and cerebral cortex (conscious perception) where it is further integrated and acted upon.

Muscle Contraction

Fig. 9-9. Components of a striated muscle cell. Each striated muscle cell (muscle fiber) contains hundreds or thousands of **myofibrils** (the number depending partly

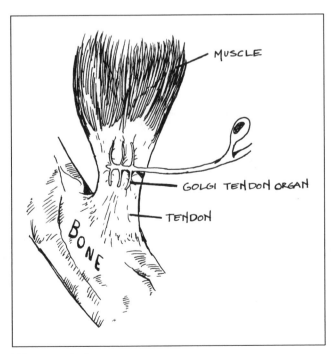

Figure 9-8

on the muscle type, but also on the degree of exercise, which causes muscle hypertrophy through increasing the number of myofibrils in the muscle cell). Each myofibril contains a series of interlocking **actin and myosin filaments**.

The **H** band is the center of the myosin filaments.

The **A** band is the entire length of the myosin filaments.

The **Z** disc is the center, and attachment site, of the actin filaments.

The **I** band encompasses the entire length of the actin filaments except for the portions that overlap the myosin filaments.

The mnemonic is "**HAZI**." The **H** band is surrounded by the **A** band; the **Z** disc is surrounded by the **I** band. A **sarcomere** is the interval between two Z discs.

Fig. 9-10. The major events in striated muscle contraction. Muscle cell contraction occurs when the actin and myosin filaments slide against one another. This process requires ATP for energy. The muscle cell contains many mitochondria, important sites of ATP production, which are interspersed between the myofibrils. Infoldings of the cell membrane, called **T tubules** (transverse tubules), are invaginations of the muscle cell membrane. These invaginations allows penetration of the electrical membrane discharge to the inner core of the muscle cell. The cell also contains a **sarcoplasmic reticulum**, an elaborate endoplasmic reticulum network which contains a high concentration of calcium. Calcium release from the sarcoplasmic reticulum is the key element that triggers the movement of the actin and myosin filaments. The release of calcium from the sacroplasmic reticulum is triggered by changes in the electric membrane potential of the muscle cell, as relayed through the T tubules. Stimuli that cause these action potentials may be mechanical, electrical, or, usually, chemical—the release of **acetylcholine** by motor nerve endings where they connect on the muscle cell (the **motor end plate**).

The mechanism of contraction of cardiac muscle is similar to that of skeletal muscle, but there is a significant difference in the utilization of calcium. In cardiac muscle, as in skeletal muscle, calcium is released from the sarcoplasmic reticulum. In addition, calcium from the interstitial fluid surrounding cardiac muscle cells enters the T tubules and from there enters the cell's cytoplasm (sarcoplasm) when the action potential spreads to the T tubules.

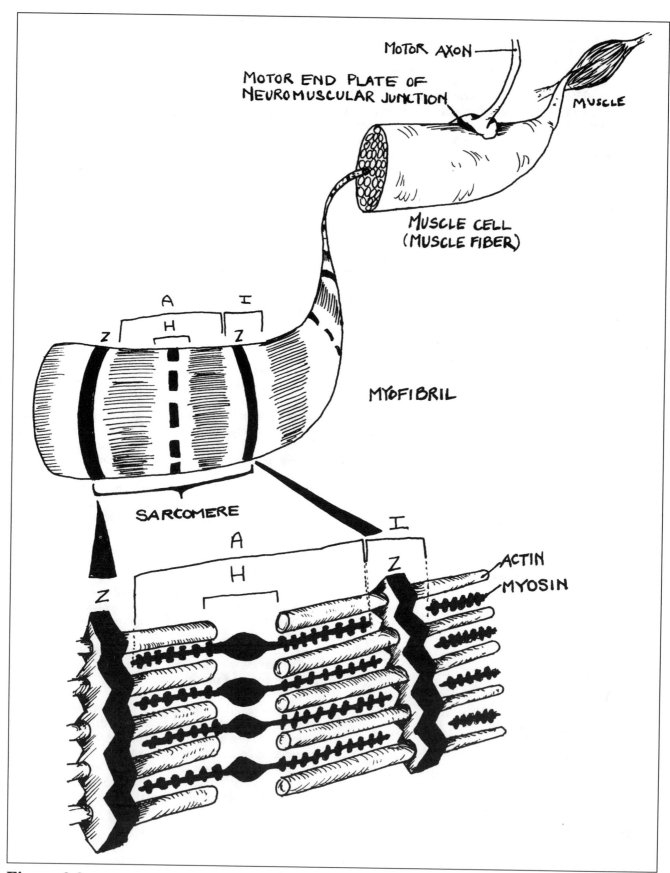

Figure 9-9

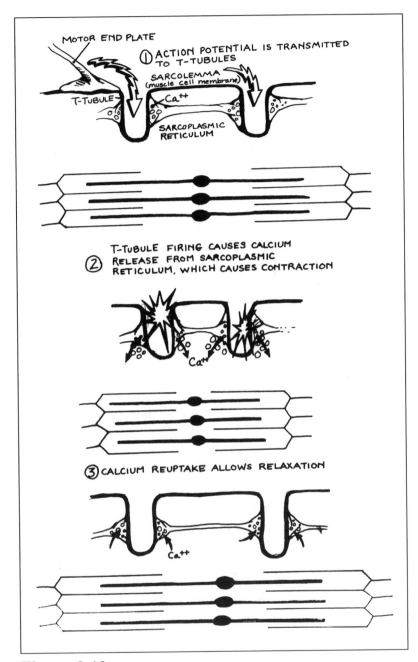

Figure 9-10

When a peripheral nerve axon divides, its branches end on a number of muscles fibers. The axon and the muscle fibers with which it connects are collectively called a **motor unit**. Many motor units fire in a given muscle action. The receptor sites for motor nerve endings on each skeletal muscle cell lie near the cell center. Hence, the action potential generated by the nerve fibers spreads in both directions to the ends of the muscle cell.

Acetylcholinesterase, an enzyme in the synaptic space of the neuromuscular junction, inactivates acetylcholine, thus preventing the prolonged and excessive action of acetylcholine on the muscle cell during a single muscle cell firing. Multiple successive contractions of a muscle's fibers can, however, be summed into a single, strong, continuous contraction called **tetany**, through the rapidly repetitive discharge of motor fibers to the muscle. The strength of the contraction may be further increased by increasing the number of motor fibers that discharge simultaneously.

The striated appearance of striated muscle is due to the geometric alignment of groups of myofibrils. Smooth muscle cells do not have this geometric alignment, but do use a modified actin-myosin interaction.

In assessing the various kinds of motor weakness, it is important to determine whether the problem lies within the nervous system or within the muscles themselves. Sometimes weakness is based on a problem within the central nervous system motor pathways, e.g. injury to a cerebral hemisphere or spinal cord motor pathway (upper motor neuron deficits). At other times weakness is due to peripheral nerve injury (lower motor neuron deficits).

Weakness may also originate with a defect at the neuromuscular junction. **Myasthenia gravis**, for instance, is an autoimmune disease which attacks the acetylcholine transport proteins at the neuromuscular junction, resulting in profound weakness. It may be treated with acetylcholinesterase inhibitors, which allow the acetylcholine that has been released into the synaptic space to stay around longer and thus act more effectively.

A defect in the plasma membrane (sarcolemma) of the striated muscle cell may cause weakness, either through unresponsiveness to stimulation (as occurs in **periodic paralysis**) or hyperresponsiveness to stimulation (as occurs in **myotonia**, where there is increased muscle contractility in an activity such as gripping an object, with difficulty in releasing the grip). In **Duchenne muscular dystrophy** there is a hereditary defect in **dystrophin**, a membrane protein necessary for the integrity of the sarcolemma.

Weakness may also result from deficits inside the muscle cell, which interfere with the normal contractile mechanism of the muscle cell.

The proper diagnosis of such conditions lies in part in sorting through the different clinical manifestation of the patient. (See Fig. 9-12 for a summary of the differences in upper versus lower motor neuron weakness). One may also find nerve and muscle biopsies helpful.

The **electromyogram (EMG)** and the testing of **nerve conduction velocities** may provide important clues as to the cause of weakness. In testing nerve conduction velocities, one electrically stimulates a periph-eral nerve, thereby simultaneously firing many nerve fibers. One then determines how long it takes for the grouped action potential to reach some distant point either along the nerve, or in its end point. If the peripheral nerve is intact, the **conduction velocity** and **amplitude** of the action potential should be normal. The amplitude of the potential will be decreased, however, in conditions where peripheral nerve fibers have been lost. Also, the nerve conduction velocity will be decreased in certain intrinsic peripheral nerve diseases (**peripheral neuropathies**).

The EMG is an important complimentary test to nerve conduction velocitiy. A needle is inserted into the muscle that is undergoing testing. There are a variety of ways to gather information in this setting; one is to have the patient contract the muscle. In myopathies, since muscle fibers have disappeared, there may be lower amplitude motor unit spike responses on attempting a contraction of a given strength. Since there are fewer muscle fibers the patient has to try harder to contract the muscle, and does so by firing more motor units, to compensate for the decrease in number of muscle fibers in each motor unit. Thus the EMG may show high frequency, low amplitude discharges in myopathies.

On the other hand, the motor unit spikes may **increase** in amplitude in peripheral nerve disease, where some nerve fibers disappear, but others may sprout and spread to take over the vacated areas on denervated muscle fibers. This expands the breadth of the persisting motor units and may cause an increased amplitude of motor unit discharge.

The hyperexcitable muscle membrane in myotonia shows rapid-firing action potentials. Muscle fibers that have been denervated exhibit slow, repetitious action potentials, called **fibrillations** (as opposed to the macroscopic, visible twitching of denervated muscles, called **fasciculations**).

NEUROANATOMY REVIEW

The following describes the general principles of neuroanatomical organization within the central nervous system, but a detailed review of neuroanatomy is beyond the scope of this book.

Fig. 9-11. Schematic view of the general flow of information in the major motor and sensory pathways. The only motor pathway shown is the corticospinal tract. One should bear in mind that other motor pathways that are functionally quite important—the so-called "extrapyramidal" pathways (tectospinal, reticulospinal, vestibulospinal, rubrospinal tracts) are not shown, for clinical simplification. The terminology is more readily

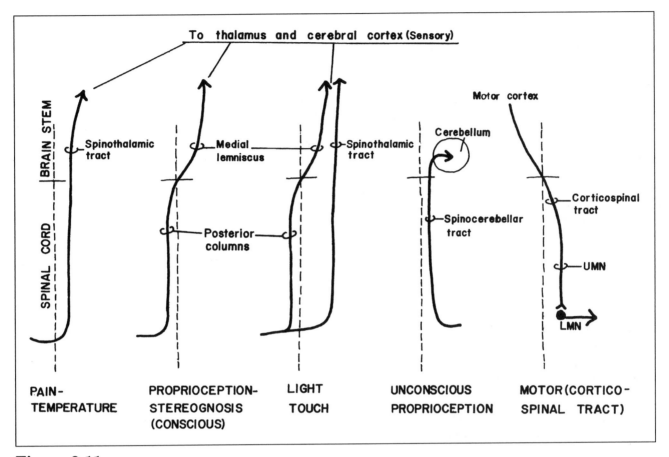

Figure 9-11

understood by realizing that the first half of a pathway name commonly refers to where the pathway originates and the latter half refers to where the pathway terminates. E.g. the spinothalamic tract originates in the spinal cord and ends in the thalamus.

As may be seen in the figure, a lesion (injury) of the pain-temperature pathway (**spinothalamic tract**), whether within the brain stem or spinal cord, results in loss of pain-temperature sensation contralaterally (i.e. on the opposite side of the body), below the level of the lesion.

A lesion at the spinal level of the pathway for conscious proprioception (the ability to sense the position and movement of the limbs) and stereognosis (the ability to identify objects by touch) results in loss of these senses ipsilaterally (i.e. on the same side) below the level of the lesion. A unilateral lesion at the brain stem level or above results in contralateral loss of conscious proprioception.

The path for light touch combines features of these two pathways. Consequently, light touch commonly is spared in unilateral spinal cord lesions because there are alternate routes to carry the information.

All of these sensory pathways eventually cross the midline, synapse in the thalamus and terminate in the sensory area of the cerebrum. Therefore, a lesion of the sensory area of the cerebral cortex results in contralateral deficits in pain-temperature, proprioception, stereognosis, and light touch sensation.

Proprioception has a conscious and an unconscious component. The conscious pathway goes to the thalamus and cerebral cortex, enabling one to describe the position of a limb. The unconscious pathway (**spinocerebellar tract**) connects with the cerebellum, which is considered an unconscious organ, and enables one to walk and perform other complex acts without having to think about which joints to flex and extend. Unlike the other sensory pathways, which cross contralaterally, the spinocerebellar tract primarily remains ipsilateral. In general, one side of the cerebellum influences the same side of the body. Thus, cerebellar lesions tend to produce ipsilateral malfunction, typically presenting as **ataxia** (awkwardness of movement), whereas cerebral lesions result in contralateral defects, manifested by weakness or sensory loss.

The corticospinal tract and related motor pathways synapse in the spinal cord, just before leaving the cord. This anatomic feature is important because motor neurons above the level of this synapse are **upper motor neurons (UMN)**, whereas the peripheral nerve cell bodies in the anterior horn of the cord, and their axonal extensions outside the cord are **lower motor neurons (LMN)**. Upper and lower motor neuron injuries produce different clinical signs. Although lesions at either level result in weakness, the presentations differ.

Fig. 9-12. Upper motor neuron (UMN) versus lower motor neuron (LMN) lesions.

Cranial nerve functions:

CN1 (Olfactory): Smells
CN2 (Optic): Sees
CNs 3,4,6 (Oculomotor, Trochlear, Abducens): Move eyes; CN3 constricts pupils, accommodates
CN5 (Trigeminal): Chews and feels front of head
CN7 (Facial): Moves the face, tastes, salivates, cries
CN8 (Vestibulocochlear): Hears, regulates balance
CN9 (Glossopharyngeal): Tastes, salivates, swallows, monitors carotid body and sinus
C10 (Vagus): Tastes, swallows, lifts palate, talks, communication to and from thoraco-abdominal viscera
CN11 (Accessory): Turns head, lifts shoulders
CN12 (Hypoglossal): Moves tongue

An injury to one side of the brain stem that affects the corticospinal tract, spinothalamic tract, or medial lemniscus will cause contralateral neurologic deficits in the extremities, in view of the crossing over of pathways, illustrated in Fig. 9-11. The same injury, if it encompasses an exiting cranial nerve, will cause ipsilateral deficits along the distribution of the affected cranial nerve. In fact, any time a patient presents with the combination of an extremity defect of any type on one side of the body and a cranial nerve deficit on the other side, one must be highly suspect that the lesion is in the brain stem.

Cerebral Lesions

A unilateral cerebral cortex lesion commonly results in weakness and sensory loss in the contralateral extremities. There may also be contralateral deficits in certain cranial nerve functions. However, unilateral cerebral cortex lesions do not affect all cranial nerves, because of **bilateral representation of function**. That is, one side of the cerebrum, rather than just connecting with cranial nerves on the opposite side of the body, connects with most cranial nerves on both sides of the body. Therefore, a lesion to one side of the cerebrum will cause little, if any, deficit, in certain cranial nerve functions, because connections from the other side of the cerebrum maintain function. For example, hoarseness may occur with a lesion of the 10th cranial nerve (vagus) but will not result from a unilateral cerebral lesion. Deafness many occur with a lesion to the cochlear nerve, but will not occur with a unilateral cerebral lesion.

Cerebral lesions do affect the cranial nerves as follows:

Olfactory Nerve (CN1). This nerve does not cross the midline. Consequently, a unilateral cortical lesion results in ipsilateral anosmia (loss of sense of smell).

Optic (CN2), Oculomotor (CN3), Trochlear (CN4) and Abducens (CN6) Nerves. Destruction of a cerebral hemisphere does not result in visual loss or ocular paralysis that is confined to the contralateral eye. Rather, both eyes are partially affected. Neither eye can move to the contralateral side (the eyes "look toward the lesion"), and neither eye sees the contralateral environment. (Mechanisms are explained in Figs. 9-13 and 9-17.)

Trigeminal Nerve (CN5). A cerebral lesion results in loss of sensation on the opposite side of the face.

Facial Nerve (CN7). Cerebral lesions generally only result in paralysis of the lower half of the face (below the eye) contralaterally, due to the strictly contralateral connections from each cerebral hemisphere to the opposite lower face. The upper face usually is not significantly involved in unilateral cerebral lesions, such as a cerebral stroke, because of bilateral connections to the forehead and eyelids from each hemisphere. The patient can raise his eyelids and close his eyes. When the facial nerve itself is damaged, as in **Bell's palsy**, there is total ipsilateral hemifacial paralysis, including the forehead and the eyelids; the patient cannot raise the eyebrow or close the eyelids on the side of the nerve lesion.

Vestibulocochlear Nerve (CN8). Hearing deficits result from local lesions between the ear and the brain-

Upper MN Defect	Lower MN Defect
spastic paralysis	flaccid paralysis
no significant muscle atrophy	significant atrophy
fasciculations and fibrillations not present	fasciculations and fibrillations present
hyperreflexia	hyporeflexia
Babinski reflex may be present	Babinski reflex not present

Figure 9-12

stem. A lesion in one hemisphere results in little deficit, because auditory information from each ear is represented bilaterally. That is, auditory fibers, upon entering the brainstem, immediately divide into ipsilateral and contralateral routes that go to both cerebral hemispheres.

Glossopharyngeal (CN9), Vagus (CN10), Accessory (CN11) and Hypoglossal (CN12) Nerves. Except for CN12, these nerves usually are not significantly affected by unilateral cerebral lesions. However, weakness of one half of the tongue may sometimes occur with a contralateral cerebral lesion, but is more striking with a direct lesion of CN12.

Fig. 9-13. The visual pathways seen from above. Optic fibers temporal (lateral) to the fovea connect with the brain ipsilaterally. Fibers nasal to the fovea cross over to the opposite side at the optic chiasm. A lesion of the optic tract on the left, therefore, results in loss of the right visual field in each eye.

Fig. 9-14. Lateral view of the visual pathways. Note (Fig. 9-13) that the right visual field falls on the left half of each retina. The superior visual field falls on the inferior retina. The right visual field projects to the left side of the brain. Similarly, the superior visual field projects below the calcarine fissure in the occipital lobe. In other words, everything is upside down and backwards, provided you think in terms of visual fields. For example, a patient with a lesion inferior to the right calcarine fissure will experience a left superior field defect (Figs. 9-13, 9-14).

The center of the retina (the fovea) projects to the tips of the occipital lobe (Fig. 9-14). Thus, a patient with a severe blow to the back of the head may experience bilateral central **scotomas** (visual field defects) if both occipital poles are destroyed. This fortunately is extremely rare.

Fig. 9-15. Pathway for the pupillary reflexes to light and accommodation. The pupillary light reflex is consensual; that is, light information from one eye reaches

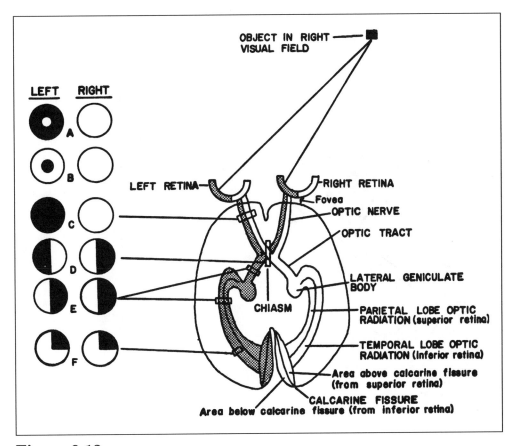

Figure 9-13

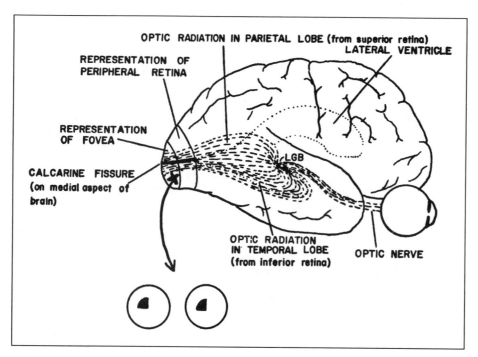

Figure 9-14

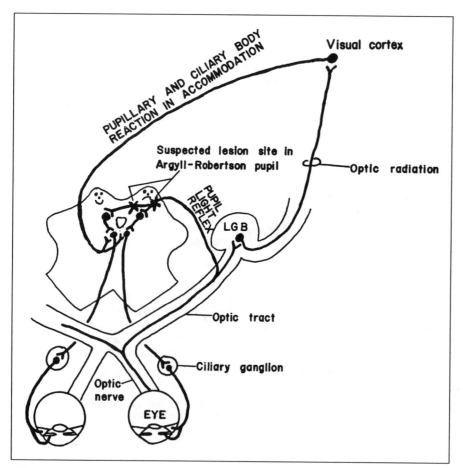

Figure 9-15

the brainstem via CN2 and returns to both eyes via CN3 on **each** side, causing both pupils to constrict. This is a brainstem-mediated reflex; cerebral lesions do not eliminate it.

Unlike the pathways mediating vision, which involve a synapse in the lateral geniculate body, the pupillary light reflex involves a direct pathway to the midbrain from the optic tract (Fig. 9-15). Shining a light in one eye normally leads to constriction of both pupils (termed the **consensual reflex**) as may be deduced from the connections depicted in Fig. 9-15. In severe optic nerve disease there will be no pupillary response when light is shined in the affected eye. There will be a consensual response when light is shined in the normal eye.

Fig. 9-16. The changes in the pupillary light reflex following CN2 or CN3 injury.

Accommodation (Fig. 9-15) involves a neural circuit to the visual cortex and back, which makes sense, for we need our cerebral cortex to determine that something is out of focus before we can send directions to correct the focus. Focusing occurs by stimulating the smooth muscle of the ciliary body in the eye to contract, thereby enabling the lens to spring back into a more spherical shape (accommodation). During accommodation not only does the lens focus but the pupils constrict, smooth muscle actions mediated by parasympathetic components of cranial nerve 3.

The syphilitic (**Argyll-Robertson**) pupil (also called the prostitute's pupil because it accommodates but does not react) constricts during accommodation, which is normal, but does not react to light. The lesion is considered to lie in the pretectal area of the superior colliculus of the midbrain (Fig. 9-15). The condition is usually bilateral. The pupils characteristically are small and somewhat irregular.

Fig. 9-17. The pathway for lateral conjugate gaze.

Damage to the motor areas of the cerebral cortex produces contralateral paralysis of the extremities. It does not produce loss of all the movements of the contralateral eye, but rather impaired ability of either eye to look voluntarily toward the contralateral environment (impairment of lateral conjugate gaze). Following a lesion to the left visuomotor area of the cerebrum, the patient cannot look to the right. Her eyes tend to deviate to the left. In essence, the eyes "look at the lesion." This occurs because the pathway from the left hemisphere innervates the right lateral rectus muscle (right CN6) and the left medial rectus muscle (left CN3). The right lateral rectus and left medial rectus muscles both direct the eyes to the right.

The Autonomic Nervous System and Hypothalamus

The autonomic system regulates glands, smooth muscle and cardiac muscle. It contains sympathetic and parasympathetic components. The sympathetic system as a whole is a catabolic system, expending energy, as in the flight or fight response to danger, e.g. increasing the heart rate and contractility and shunting blood to the muscles and heart. The parasympathetic system is an anabolic system, conserving energy, e.g. in slowing the heart rate and in promoting the digestion and absorption of food. The cell bodies of preganglionic sympathetic fibers lie in the intermediolateral columns of the spinal cord at spinal cord level T1-L2 (Fig. 9-19). Those of the parasympathetic system occupy comparable positions at spinal cord levels S2-S4. In addition, cranial nerves 3,7, 9, and 10 have parasympathetic components (3—pupil and ciliary body constriction; 7—tearing and salivation; 9—salivation; 10—the vagus and its ramifications).

Fig. 9-18. A. The sympathetic nerve routes. B. The parasympathetic nerve routes.

	Right CN3 Lesion	Right CN2 Lesion
Light shined in right eye	Only left pupil constricts	No pupil constricts
Light shined in left eye	Only left pupil constricts	Both pupils constrict

Figure 9-16

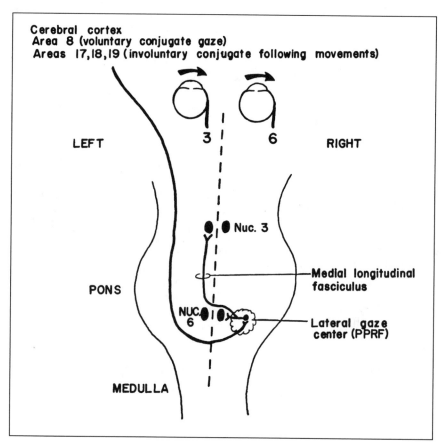

Figure 9-17

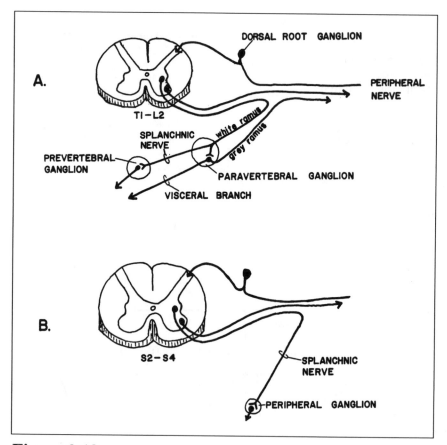

Figure 9-18

In order to extend all over the body, the sympathetic system fibers leave the spinal cord at cord levels T1-L2, enter the paravertebral ganglion chain and then may travel up or down the chain for considerable distances prior to synapsing (Fig. 9-19). The sympathetic chain stretches from the foramen magnum to the coccyx and supplies the far reaches of the body with post-ganglionic sympathetic fibers. Parasympathetic fibers reach widespread areas via the vagus (Fig. 9-19).

Fig. 9-19. Schematic view of the autonomic nervous system.

Both parasympathetic and sympathetic systems contain two neurons between the spinal cord and periphery. The first synapse is cholinergic (containing acetylcholine). For the sympathetic system, this synapse is either in the paravertebral chain of sympathetic ganglia or farther away in the prevertebral ganglion plexuses (Fig. 9-18).

Parasympathetic synapses typically lie very close to or within the viscera. The final synapse of the parasympathetic system contains acetylcholine, whereas the final synapse of the sympathetic system contains norepinephrine, with the exception of certain synapses, as for sweating, that contain acetylcholine (i.e. are cholinergic). In the chart below, note that secretory actions in general are stimulated by cholinergic fibers.

Fig. 9-20. Sympathetic and parasympathetic functions.

In extreme fear, both systems may act simultaneously, producing involuntary emptying of the bladder and rectum (parasympathetic) along with a generalized sympathetic response. In more pleasant circumstances, namely in sexual arousal, the parasympathetic system mediates penile and clitoral erection and the sympathetic controls ejaculation. (You can remember the difference, as "parasympathetic" is a longer word.)

Proceeding rostrally from the caudal tip of the spinal cord, one first finds a parasympathetic area (S2-S4), followed by a sympathetic region (T1-L2), then parasympathetic areas (CNs 10, 9, 7, 3) and then successively a sympathetic and a parasympathetic area, a strange alternating sequence. The latter two areas are the posterior and anterior parts of the hypothalamus (Fig. 9-19).

The hypothalamus, a structure about the size of a thumbnail, is the master control for the autonomic system. Stimulation or lesions result not in isolated smooth muscle, cardiac muscle or glandular effects but in organized actions involving these systems, e.g. in the fear or rage reaction of the flight or fight response, in increased and decreased appetite, altered sexual functioning, and control of body temperature. For instance, stimulation of the posterior hypothalamus may result in conservation of body heat and an increase in body temperature owing to constriction of cutaneous blood vesels.

Many circuits connect the hypothalamus with various areas of the cerebral cortex, brain stem and thalamus.

Fig. 9-21. The reverberating **Papez circuit** (modified from Manter and Gatz's ESSENTIALS OF CLINICAL NEUROANATOMY AND NEUROPHYSIOLOGY, by S. Gilman and S. Winans Newman, 7th Edition, 1987), believed to be involved in the emotional content of conscious thought processes. It provides intercommunication between hippocampus, hypothalamus, thalamus and cerebral cortex. Note the input of the olfactory system, which also plays a role in emotion. This is evident if you have ever seen two dogs sniffing one another or noted the prominence of the perfume industry in major department stores.

In **Wernicke's syndrome**, which occurs in patients who are alcoholic and undernourished, there is paralysis of eye movements, ataxic gait and disturbances in the state of consciousness associated with hemorrhages in the hypothalamus and other regions. **Korsakoff's syndrome** also occurs in alcoholic patients and consists of memory loss, confusion and confabulation associated with lesions in the mammillary bodies and associated areas. (The mammillary bodies are considered a part of the hypothalamus.)

Fig. 9-22. The major connections between hypothalamus and pituitary gland. The hypothalamus lies close to the pituitary gland. A disorder of one structure may affect the other. Note that nerve fibers from the paraventricular and supraoptic nuclei connect with the posterior pituitary. These nuclei secrete **oxytocin**

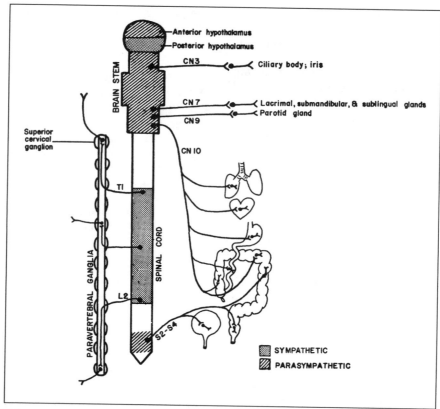

Figure 9-19

and **antidiuretic hormone (vasopressin)**. These hormones are synthesized and transported in neurons and then released at the ends of the nerve terminals in the posterior pituitary.

The anterior pituitary contains no neuronal connections. Instead, releasing factors are produced in the hypothalamus and are released into the portal circulation and then transported to the anterior pituitary where they stimulate cells in the anterior pituitary to secrete various hormones, including adrenocorticotrophic hormone, thyrotrophic hormone, somatotrophic hormone, follicle stimulating hormone and luteininzing hormone. These are described in greater detail in the Endocrine chapter.

In a sense, the pituitary hormones are involved in autonomic-type functions, but on a more prolonged time scale. For instance, thyroid hormone is catabolic; growth hormone is anabolic; FSH, LH, and oxytocin relate to sexual functioning, and antidiuretic hormone relates to blood pressure.

Disorders of the autonomic system include:

1) **Riley-Day syndrome (familial dysautonomia)**, a disease associated with degenerative changes in the central nervous system and the peripheral autonomic system. Symptoms include decreased lacrimation, transient skin blotching, attacks of hypertension, episodes of hyperpyrexia and vomiting, impairment of taste discrimination, relative insensitivity to pain, and emotional instability.

2) **Adiposogenital syndrome**, characterized by obesity and retarded development of secondary sexual characteristics, sometimes is associated with lesions in the hypothalmus.

3) **Precocious puberty** may result from hypothalamic tumors.

4) The **common cold**. Temperature elevation is apparently the consequence of an influence on hypothalamic functioning.

5) Tumors of the pituitary may have a destructive effect on the pituitary gland and hypothalamus by direct extension, e.g. in chromophobe adenoma and craniopharyngioma, which generally are nonsecretory tumors. If the tumor contains functioning glandular tissue, e.g. acidophilic or basophilic adenoma, there may be the opposite effect of hypersecretion of pituitary hormones.

Structure	Sympathetic function	Parasympathetic function
Eye	Dilates pupil (mydriasis) No significant effect on ciliary muscle	Contracts pupil (miosis) Contracts ciliary muscle (accommodation)
Lacrimal gland	No significant effect	Stimulates secretion
Salivary glands	No significant effect	Stimulates secretion
Sweat glands	Stimulates secretion (cholinergic fibers)	No significant effect
Heart Rate	Increases	Decreases
Force of ventricular contraction	Increases	Decreases
Blood vessels	Dilates or constricts cardiac & skeletal muscle vessels* Constricts skin and digestive system blood vessels	No significant effect
Lungs	Dilates bronchial tubes	Constricts bronchial tubes Stimulates bronchial gland secretion
Gastrointestinal tract	Inhibits motility and secretion	Stimulates motility and secretion
GI sphincters	contracts	relaxes
Adrenal medulla	Stimulates secretion of adrenaline (cholinergic fibers)	No significant effect
Urinary bladder	?	Contracts
Sex organs	Ejaculation	Erection

*Stimulation of beta-2 receptors *dilates* cardiac and skeletal muscle, whereas stimulation of alpha-1 receptors *constricts*. Most dilation of cardiac and skeletal vessels, though, may be due to non-autonomic, local tissue *autoregulatory* responses to lack of oxygen.

Figure 9-20

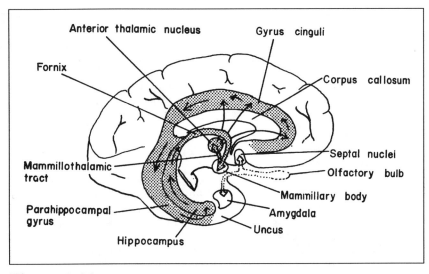

Figure 9-21

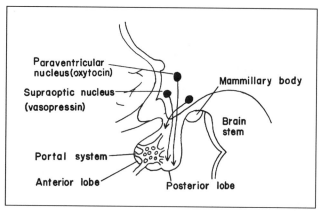

Figure 9-22

6) **Diabetes insipidus.** Vasopressin (antidiuretic hormone) enhances the reuptake of water in the kidney. Interference with its production, as by an invading tumor, leads to diabetes insipidus, characterized by excessive production of urine and excessive thirst.

7) **Horner's syndrome.** Interruption of the cervical sympathetic nerves (or in some cases their central origins in the spinal cord and brain stem) leads to ptosis, miosis and decrease in sweating on the involved side of the face. Sometimes this is the result of a tumor of the apex of the lung (Pancoast tumor) that interrupts the fibers as they course from the superior cervical ganglion (the most rostral ganglion in the sympathetic chain) to the carotid artery on their way to the orbit.

8) **Hirschprung's megacolon.** There is congenital absence of parasympathetic ganglion cells in the wall of the colon, resulting in poor colonic motility and a dilated colon.

Cerebellum, Basal Ganglia, and Thalamus

Clinically, it is not very important to know the complex internal connections of the thalamus, cerebellum and basal ganglia, and these will not be emphasized.

The Thalamus

The thalamus is a sensory relay and integrative center connecting with many areas of the brain, including the cerebral cortex, basal ganglia, hypothalamus and brain stem. It is capable of perceiving pain but not of accurate localization. For instance, patients with tumors of the thalamus may experience the "thalamic pain syndrome," a vague sense of pain without the ability to accurately localize it. Sensory fibers, ascending through the brain stem, synapse in the thalamus and are then relayed to the cerebral cortex via the internal capsule.

Motor fibers descending from the cortex pass to the brain stem via the internal capsule without synapsing in the thalamus. Fig. 9-23 illustrates the anatomy of this region.

The lentiform nucleus (the putamen plus globus pallidus) lies lateral to the internal capsule, whereas the caudate nucleus and thalamus lie medial. Note in Fig. 9-23 the distribution of head, arm, and leg fibers in the internal capsule.

Fig. 9-23. The internal capsule and its relationship to the caudate nucleus (C), thalamus (T), and lentiform nucleus (L). A. Lateral view. B. Horizontal section at the level indicated in A. C. Cross section at the level indicated in A. D. The course of the major motor and sensory pathways. H, head; A, arm; L, leg.

The Cerebellum and Basal Ganglia

Rather than list the multitude of complex cerebellar and basal ganglia connections, it is clinically more important to understand the types of clinical syndromes that may occur in these two systems. In general, cerebellar dysfunction is characterized by awkwardness of intentional movements. Basal ganglia disorders are more characterized by meaningless unintentional movements occurring unexpectedly.

Cerebellar Disorders

1) Ataxia—awkwardness of posture and gait; tendency to fall to the same side as the cerebellar lesion; poor coordination of movement; overshooting the goal in reaching toward an object (**dysmetria**); inability to perform rapid alternating movements (**dysdiadochokinesia**), such as finger tapping; scanning speech due to awkward use of speech muscles, resulting in irregularly spaced sounds.
2) Decreased tendon reflexes on the affected side.
3) Asthenia—muscles tire more easily than normal
4) Tremor—usually an intention tremor (evident during purposeful movements).
5) Nystagmus (a repetitive, tremor-like oscillating movement of the eyes).

Basal Ganglia Disorders

1) **Parkinsonism**—rigidity; slowness; resting tremor; mask-like facies; shuffling gait, associated with degeneration in the basal ganglia and substantia nigra.
2) **Chorea**—sudden jerky and purposeless movements (e.g. Syndenham's chorea found in rheumatic fever; Huntington's chorea, an inherited disorder).
3) **Athetosis**—slow writhing, snake-like movements, especially of the fingers and wrists.

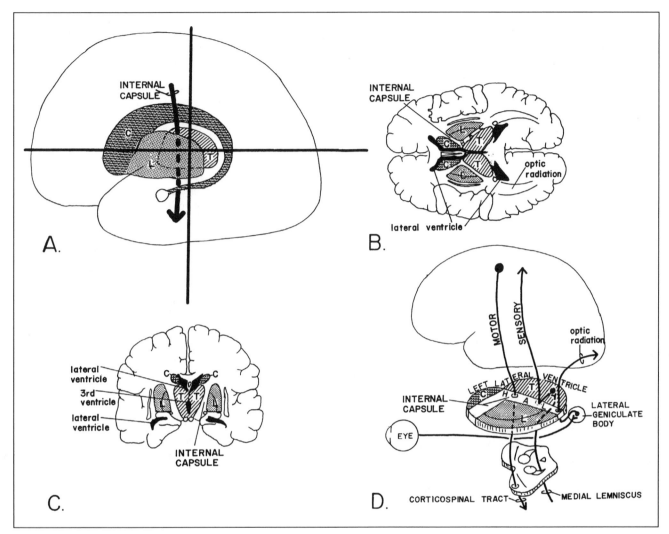

Figure 9-23

4) **Hemiballismus**—a sudden wild flail-like movement of one arm.

Cerebral Cortex

Lesions to the nervous system may lead to simple or complex levels of dysfunction depending upon the area involved. For instance, if one asks a patient to put on a polo shirt and his left brachial plexus is severed, he will only use his right arm, as his left arm is paralyzed. The cerebellum and basal ganglia represent a step further in levels of functioning. With a cerebellar lesion, the patient may perform the act awkwardly, e.g. overshooting the mark, or with tremor. With basal ganglia lesions there may be unexpected, unplanned totally irrelevant movements, beyond the realm of awkwardness, e.g. a sudden flail-like movement, etc. In the cerebral cortex,

unless the lesion is in the primary motor area wherein paralysis may result, a higher level of dysfunction may be found, e.g. the patient trying to get his head into the sleeve or trying other inadequate orientations.

In speech, a lesion of CN10 may result in hoarseness (laryngeal dysfunction). When cranial nerves 10, 12 or 7 are involved, there may be difficulty with the "KLM" sounds; i.e. the sounds "Kuh, Kuh, Kuh" test the soft palate (CN10), "LA, LA, LA," the tongue (CN12) and "MI, MI, MI" the lips (CN7). With lesions in the speech areas of the cerebral cortex, the deficit may involve higher levels of speech organization—the deletion of words or inclusion of excessive or inappropriate words. In psychiatric disturbances, the level of dysfunction is even higher with abnormalitites in the entire pattern of thought organization.

It is similar for the sensory pathways. Simple anesthesia (total sensory loss) may result from lesions between the primary sensory cortex and the body periphery. In other brain areas, the patient may have difficulty in comprehending the incoming information. For instance, a lesion to the optic tract results in homonymous hemianopia (neither eye can see the environment contralateral to the lesion). In lesions to cortical areas 18 and 19 the patient sees but may not recognize what he is looking at.

Complex cerebral receptive disabilities are called **agnosias**. Complex cerebral motor disabilities are **apraxias**. Often the two are difficult to distinguish.

When language function is involved, the disabilities are termed **aphasias**. Aphasia may be receptive (i.e. reading, listening) or motor (i.e. writing, talking). For aphasia to occur, the lesion must be in the dominant hemisphere, which is the left hemisphere in right handed people and in many (but not all) left handed people.

Fig. 9-24. Major regions of the cerebrum. The shaded area indicates the region of the cerebral cortex involved with aphasia. Subdivisions of this area are logical. Lesions in the anterior part of this area, near the motor cortex, tend to result in expressive aphasia. Lesions more posterior, near the auditory and visual cortex, result in receptive aphasia. Lesions nearer the visual cortex result in inability to read (**alexia**). Lesions near the auditory cortex result in inability to understand speech. Actually, difficulty in talking may result from both anterior or posterior lesions. Following lesions in the more anterior regions of the aphasic zone, speech disturbances tend to be nonfluent; the patient omits nouns and connector words like **but**, **or** and **and**. In the more posterior regions his words are plentiful or even excessive, but he crams into his speech inappropriate word substitutes, circumlocutions and neologisms—a word salad. Presumably, this is because the ability to speak also depends on the ability to understand what one is saying. Thus, if the aphasic area near the auditory cortex is involved, this will also result in a defect in speech.

Lesions to corresponding areas of the non-dominant hemisphere do not result in aphasia, but rather in visual or auditory inattention to the left environment or to general unawareness of the concept of "left." The patient may deny he has any neurological deficit despite a dense hemiplegia and left visual field defect.

Specific cerebral cortical regions and the effects of lesions are listed below.

Area 4 (the primary motor area). Lesions result in initial flaccid paralysis followed in several months by partial recovery of function and a possible Babinski reflex; spasticity and increased deep tendon reflexes may occur if area 6 (the supplemental motor area) is included.

Lesions to **area 8 (the frontal eye fields)** result in difficulty in voluntarily moving the eyes to the opposite side.

Areas of the frontal cortex rostral to the motor area are involved in complex behavioral activites. Lesions result in changes in judgement, abstract thinking, tactfulness and foresight. Symptoms may include irresponsibility in dealing with daily affairs, vulgar speech and clownish behavior.

Areas 44,45 (Broca's speech area). The patient with a lesion in this area experiences motor aphasia, but only when the dominant hemisphere is involved. The patient knows what he wants to say but speech is slow, deleting many prepositions and nouns.

Areas 3,1,2 (primary somesthetic area). Lesions produce contralateral impairment of touch, pressure and proprioception. Pain sensation will be impaired if the lesion lies in the **secondary somesthetic sensory area** (Fig. 9-24) which receives pain information.

Areas 41,42 (auditory area). Unilateral lesions have little effect on hearing owing to the bilateral representation of the auditory pathways. Significant auditory defects generally involve either CN8 or its entry point in the brain stem, for bilateral representation begins beyond this point in the brain stem.

Area 22 (Wernicke's area). Lesions in the dominant hemisphere result in auditory aphasia. The patient

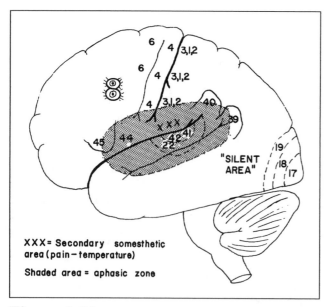

XXX= Secondary somesthetic area (pain-temperature)

Shaded area = aphasic zone

Figure 9-24

hears but does not understand. He speaks but makes mistakes unknowingly owing to his inability to understand his own words.

Area 40 (supramarginal gyrus). Lesions in the dominant hemisphere result in tactile and proprioceptive agnosia, and a variety of other problems, such as confusion in left-right discrimination, disturbances of body-image, and apraxia, by cutting off impulses to and from association tracts that interconnect this area with nearby regions.

Area 39 (angular gyrus). Lesions in the dominant hemisphere may result in alexia and agraphia (inability to read and write).

Areas 17,18, 19. Total destruction causes blindness in the contralateral visual field. Lesions to areas 18 and 19 alone do not cause blindness but rather difficulty in recognizing and identifying objects (**visual agnosia**).

The **silent area** is believed to function in memory storage of visual and auditory information and is implicated in hallucinations and dreams. Epileptic attacks originating in this region may be associated with amnesia, auditory hallucinations, and the deja vu phenomenon.

Localization of Neurologic Problems

In approaching a patient with a neurologic problem, there are a number of key questions that help establish the localization of the lesion:

1) Is there a dermatome deficit (Fig. 9-25)? If so, this suggests a peripheral nerve lesion, as the central nervous system is not organized according to dermatomes. Lesions to central nervous system sensory pathways more likely will cause a general loss of sensation in an extremity than the strip-like deficit of a dermatome lesion.

Fig. 9-25. Dermatomes, the distribution of sensory nerves on the skin.

2) Is there localized pain? Lesions to sensory areas of the central nervous system tend to cause loss of pain rather than pain itself. The presence of localized pain suggests irritation of a peripheral nerve or nerve root.

3) Are there upper or lower motor neuron signs (Fig. 9-12)? This will help pinpoint whether the lesion lies at the CNS (UMN) or peripheral nerve (LMN) level.

4) Is there a dissociation of sensory loss, i.e. loss of pain-temperature in one extremity, but loss of proprioception in the other extremity? This suggests a spinal cord lesion, because the sensory pathways cross at different levels of the spinal cord, but have all crossed (except for the spinocerebellar tract) by the time they reach the brain stem.

5) Is there cranial nerve involvement? If so, this establishes the localization of the lesion above the foramen magnum, where the spinal cord becomes the brainstem.

6) Is there some combination of a cranial nerve deficit on one side of the face, and an extremity deficit on the other side (for example, a dilated fixed pupil on the right, combined with paralysis or sensory loss of the left upper and lower extremities)? If so, this indicates a brainstem lesion, because lesions below the brainstem would not cause cranial nerve deficits, and lesions above the brain stem would cause deficits restricted to the contralateral environment.

7) Which cranial nerves are involved? If there is a unilateral loss of CN3 (pupil enlarged, unresponsive to light; failure of the eye to adduct), or unilateral loss of CN6 (failure of the eye to abduct), or facial (CN7) weakness on one **entire** side of the face (i.e. manifest in both the upper and lower face), or atrophy and fasciculations of one side of the tongue, this suggests either a brainstem injury or injury to the nerve more peripherally. Cerebral lesions would not cause such deficits, due to the bilateral innervation of these cranial nerves.

Bilateral lesions of the cerebral cortex or internal capsule (the area where cerebral cortex fibers funnel into the brainstem) may result in **pseudobulbar palsy,** in which there are multiple cranial nerve deficits. The patient then experiences difficulties with facial expression, movement of the tongue, chewing, swallowing, speech and breathing. There also may be inappropriate spells of laughing or crying as part of the syndrome.

8) Is there awkwardness of movement? Weakness in an extremity can cause awkwardness of movement, but in the absence of weakness, one must ask whether the problem lies at the cerebellar level or the basal ganglia? Awkwardness of **intended movements (ataxia)** or tremor on intended movements suggest a lesion of the cerebellum or its connecting pathways. **Involuntary movements** (e.g. resting tremor, **chorea** (uncontrolled awkward jerky movements), **athetosis** (writhing movements), **hemiballismus** (wild flinging movements of an extremity) are characteristic of basal ganglia lesions.

9) It may be difficult to differentiate a lesion in the cerebral cortex from one in the internal capsule (the region in the core of the brain where motor and sensory fibers funnel into and out of the brain stem). The presence of a higher level dysfunction suggests a cerebral cortex lesion. This may include an **agnosia** (complex receptive disability, e.g. loss of ability to understand what one is reading while retaining the ability to see), **apraxia** (complex motor disability, such as putting on one's pants backwards), and **aphasia** (complex speech disturbance, as opposed to simple hoarseness or monotone).

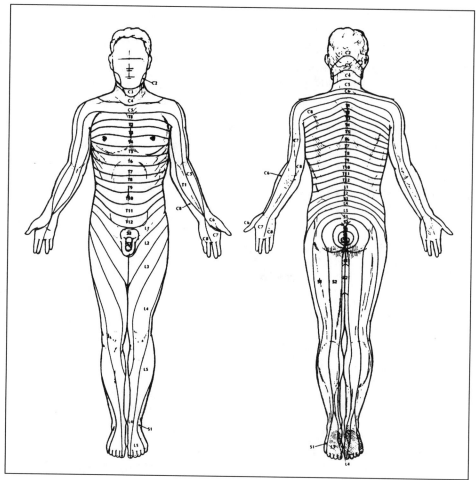

Figure 9-25

The Electroencephalogram (EEG)

The EEG is a record of the summed underlying neuronal activity of the brain, as sampled in a number of areas over the scalp.

Fig. 9-26. Normal EEG patterns. Brain waves vary in their frequency. They tend to be fastest when the subject is most alert (beta waves, >13 waves/sec (also called Hertz/second or just Hz). Alpha waves are somewhat slower (8–13Hz/sec) and occur in a state of quiet awareness, but also in the dream phase (REM, or rapid eye movement phase) of sleep. Theta waves (4–7Hz) are slower and occur in drowsiness, whereas Delta waves (<4Hz) are even slower, occurring in deep sleep or in the pathologically depressed brain. A flat EEG occurs in brain death, but can also occur in certain states of drug overdosage.

Fig. 9-27. EEG patterns in epilepsy. Analysis of the EEG can be useful diagnostically. Diffuse slowing of the

waves is often found in organic mental syndrome. Focal localization of the slowing often points to a discrete neurologic lesion, although MRI scans and other imaging procedures are generally much more useful in localizing a lesion. In epilepsy, abnormal discharges are seen on

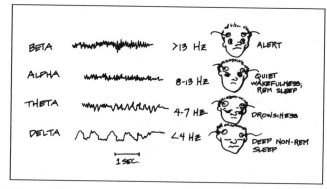

Figure 9-26

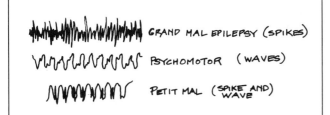

Figure 9-27

the EEG, which contains abnormal sharp waves or spikes. In **grand mal epilepsy**, there is diffuse rapid, high amplitude firing that coincides with a diffuse epileptic seizure. The patient may have shaking of the extremities, tongue biting, and urinary and fecal incontinence secondary to diffuse electrical seizure discharges. In focal ("**Jacksonian**") seizures, which involve seizures of a limited area of the body, e.g. the arm, the seizure activity is more localized, and often can be traced to a focal scar or tumor as the factor that generates the seizure. In **petit mal** epilepsy, a condition that mainly affects children, there are brief unresponsive periods of staring, along with a "spike and dome" pattern to the EEG. In **psychomotor seizures**, there may be organized patterns of uncontrollable abnormal social behavior, rather than shaking movements. **Uncinate seizures**, which originate in the uncus of the temporal lobe, are characterized by the experience of abnormal smells, such as burning rubber.

THE SPECIAL SENSES: VISION

Fig. 9-28. Sagittal section through the human eye.

It is difficult to play billiards using eyeballs, as the eye is not perfectly spherical. The cornea is too steeply curved. This steep curvature enables the cornea to perform most of the refraction (bending and focusing) of light entering the eye. The cornea provides a coarse, nonvariable focus. The lens also focuses light, but only performs the fine variable adjustments. Contact lenses artificially alter the curvature of the front of the eye, thereby changing the focus.

The eye has three chambers: the **anterior chamber (A.C.)** (in front of the iris), the **posterior chamber (P)** (between the iris and the lens), and the **vitreous chamber** (behind the lens). The anterior and posterior chambers contain the clear, watery **aqueous humor** produced constantly by the **ciliary body**. Aqueous humor (arrows) exits the eye via the circular **canal of Schlemm (S)**, which lies in the angle between the cornea and iris. The canal of Schlemm communicates directly with venous circulation. Blockage of aqueous out-

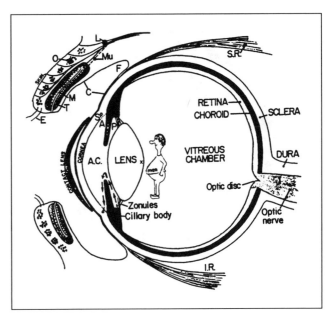

Figure 9-28

flow results in increased intraocular pressure, termed **glaucoma**.

The ciliary body not only produces aqueous humor, but also contains a ring of ciliary muscle (Fig. 9-29) that is attached to the lens via fine, ligamentous **zonule fibers**. Contraction of the ciliary muscles affects the shape of the lens, thereby changing its focus—the process of **accommodation.**

Fig. 9-29. Posterior view of the ciliary muscle ring.

The mechanism of accommodation is more easily understood by first considering the mechanism of pupillary expansion (dilation) and constriction, as follows. The iris contains circular (constrictor) muscles at the pupillary border, and radial (dilator) muscle fibers (Fig. 9-30).

Fig. 9-30. Constrictor and dilator muscles of the iris. Note how contraction of the radial fibers would dilate the pupil. Contraction of the constrictor muscles decreases the circumference of the ring; therefore, the pupil constricts. The ciliary muscles, although more complex than the iris constrictor muscles, in a sense act similarly. Contraction of muscles in the ciliary ring narrows the diameter of the ring. This decreases the tension of the zonules, and releases tension on the lens. The lens then springs back into a thicker, rounder shape leading to a stronger focus (accommodation). Thus, accommodation is the process in which the ciliary muscles contract, thereby relaxing tension on the lens and enabling one to focus closer on an object.

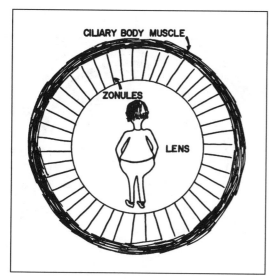

Figure 9-29

Opacities in the lens (**cataracts**) may obstruct vision, particularly when they are positioned centrally, in the posterior aspect of the lens ("x" in Fig. 9-28). For optical reasons, cataracts in the anterior aspect of the lens or at the lens periphery tend to cause less visual loss.

The vitreous chamber contains vitreous humor, a thick gel. Unlike the aqueous humor, vitreous humor is no longer produced in the mature eye. Vitreous that is lost inadvertently from the eye during intraocular surgery cannot be replaced; fortunately, normal saline or aqueous humor may be substituted.

The eye has three main coats—the **retina**, **choroid** (a very vascular, pigmented structure), and **sclera** (the

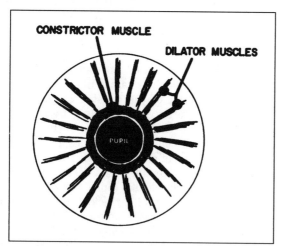

Figure 9-30

avascular "white of the eye"). After passing through the cornea, anterior chamber, pupil, posterior chamber, lens and vitreous chamber, light then strikes the transparent retina.

Fig. 9-31. Cross section through the retina. Light passes through the entire thickness of the retina before striking the photoreceptors. The photoreceptor cells initiate a chain of neuronal impulses from photoreceptor to bipolar cell to ganglion cell. (Actually the information spread through these short neurons does not occur through action potentials but by direct electron flow, as would occur in an electrical wire. Actual action potentials begin at the level of the retinal ganglion cells.) The ganglion cell axons become the optic nerve, which extends across the optic chiasm to the lateral geniculate body, from which visual fibers radiate to the visual cortex of the brain. Except for some amacrine cells which participate in the direct flow of information in the neuronal pathway from retinal photoreceptors to brain, most amacrine and horizontal cells are not part of the direct chain but do have important modifying influences on it. One of the most important of these effects is **lateral inhibition**, in which amacrine and horizontal cells inhibit the firing of cells lateral to the direct chain of neuronal communication. This prevents undue spread of electrical activity and contributes to increased visual acuity. Bipolar cells also contribute to lateral inhibition, since some of them depolarize (are stimulated) while adjacent ones hyperpolarize (are inhibited) in response to information coming from a stimulated photoreceptor.

Lateral inhibition is reflected in the activity of retinal ganglion cells. Ganglion cells typically fire continuously to some degree, with or without light stimulation. Many ganglion cells are particularly sensitive to **changes** in illumination. When light is suddenly shined in a narrow focus directly above the ganglion cell, the cell fires, while firing abruptly stops when the light is withdrawn. When the light is shined just lateral to the cell the firing pattern decreases, due to lateral inhibition, whereas the firing suddenly increases on withdrawal of the laterally-shined light. Such ganglion cells respond more vigorously to edges (detection of contrast) than to diffuse light, because the patterns of light and dark in an edge add to one another in stimulating a given ganglion cell.

Most of the retina receives its nutrition from branches of the central retinal artery, which lie within the retina. The photoreceptor cells, however, receive their nutrition largely by diffusion from the choroid. In **retinal detachment**, the retina separates from the pigment epithelium, a single layer of cells that lies closely adherent to the choroid. If not repaired with several days, the photoreceptors may be irreversibly damaged from prolonged hypoxia.

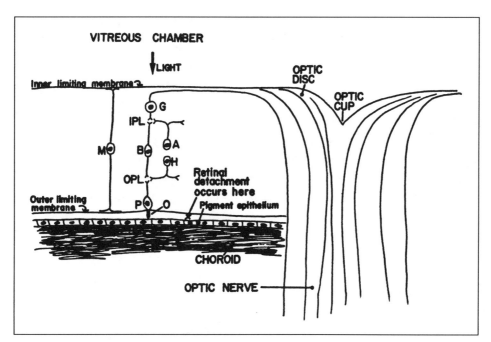

Figure 9-31 (A, Amacrine cell; B, Bipolar cell; G, Ganglion cell; H, Horizontal cell; IPL, Inner plexiform layer; M, Muller cell; O, Outer segment of photoreceptor cell; OPL, Outer plexiform layer; P, Photoreceptor cell)

"Uvea" refers to the combination of the choroid, ciliary body and iris. All these structures are pigmented and continuous with one another. If one were to remove the sclera, one would note with great shock that the entire underlying eye, not just the iris, is pigmented. **Uveitis** is an inflammation of the uvea. Uveitis is "posterior" when the choroid is involved, or "anterior" when the ciliary body or iris is involved. **Chorioretinitis** is an inflammation that affects both choroid and retina.

The Eye Muscles

Fig. 9-32. Anatomy of the extraocular eye muscles (S.O., superior oblique; I.O., inferior oblique; S.R., superior rectus; M.R., medial rectus; I.R., inferior rectus; L.R., lateral rectus). Note that each muscle attaches at one end to the eye and at the other end to some position on the nasal aspect of the orbit. None of the eye muscles attach to the temporal wall of the orbit. Keeping this in mind, you can appreciate the function of the eye muscles by imagining yourself pulling on each muscle in Fig. 9-32. The eye will move as indicated in Fig. 9-33.

Fig. 9-33. Movements of the extraocular muscles.

Refractive Disorders

If a camera is unfocused, focusing will help to sharpen the image. If the camera has a cloudy lens or damaged film, focusing will not help. Similarly, poor vi-

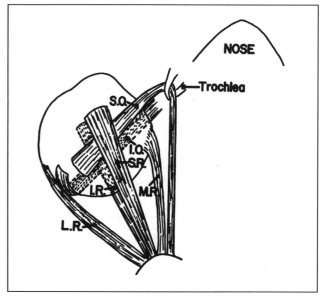

Figure 9-32

sual acuity may stem either from refractive errors (which may be improved by glasses) or from non-refractive errors, e.g. corneal opacity, cataract, retinal detachment (which glasses will not correct).

One can often distinguish refractive from non-refractive problems by determining the visual acuity at far

113

Eye Muscle	Nerve	Primary Function	Deficit
Medial rectus	Oculomotor (CN3)	Moves eye nasally	Eye is down and out because of unopposed action of lateral rectus and superior oblique
Lateral rectus	Abducens (CN6)	Moves eye temporally	Eye cannot look temporally
Superior rectus	Oculomotor (CN3)	Moves eye up	Weakness of upward gaze
Inferior rectus	Oculomotor (CN3)	Moves eye down	Weakness of downward gaze
Superior oblique	Trochlear (CN4)	1) Moves eye down when eye is already looking nasally. 2) Rotates eye when eye is already looking temporally. 3) Moves eye down and out when eye is in straight ahead position.	Vertical diplopia Head tilt (compensation for imbalance of rotation).
Inferior oblique	Oculomotor (CN3)	1) Moves eye up when eye is already looking nasally. 2) Rotates eye when eye is already looking temporally. 3) Moves eye up and out when eye is in straight ahead position.	Vertical diplopia Head tilt
Levator palpebrae superioris	Oculomotor (CN3)	Elevates upper lid	Marked ptosis
Muller's muscle (see Fig. 1)	Cervical sympathetics	Elevates upper lid	Mild ptosis

Figure 9-33

(via a Snellen chart, which is read at 20 feet away) and comparing it with that at near (via a hand-held Rosenbaum card—see Fig. 9-34). If near vision is good but not far, or vice-versa, the problem is refractive. Obviously, non-refractive problems lead to poor vision at both distances, just as a cloudy camera lens or torn film results in a poor picture regardless of the distance or focus. If vision is poor at both distances, the problem may be either refractive or non-refractive. Under such circumstances the nature of the problem may be uncovered either by testing lenses of various powers to determine whether they improve vision (a refractive rerror) or

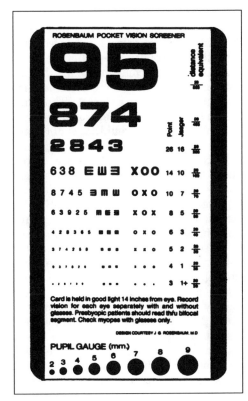

Figure 9-34

whether a pinhole improves vision (also a refractive error). The pinhole principle is illustrated in Fig. 9-35.

Fig. 9-34. The Rosenbaum hand-held vision card.

Fig. 9-35. The pinhole lens. The pinhole restricts light to the center of the cornea, where refraction (bending of the light) is unnecessary. Light remains in focus regardless of the refractive error of the eye. The next time you lose your eyeglasses in the woods, try viewing through a pinhole; vision will improve. Pinhole glasses

would be used more frequently except that they decrease both the illumination and the field of vision, in addition to the weird cosmetic appearance.

For good vision, light must focus precisely on the retina. In nearsightedness (**myopia:** the patient sees near objects best), light end up focused in front of the retina (Fig. 9-36). In far-sightedness (**hyperopia**: the patient see far objects best), light focuses behind the retina. Fig. 9-37 illustrates why myopes have greatest difficulty with far vision, whereas hyperopes have greatest difficulty with near vision.

Fig. 9-36. Myopia and hyperopia.

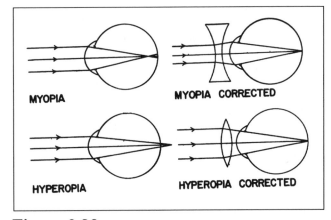

Figure 9-36

Fig. 9-37. The closer an object (o) is to a convex lens, the farther is the image (i) focused. Hence, (see Fig. 9-36) for myopes, near objects are focused closer to the retina than far objects and are seen best. For hyperopes, far objects focus closer to the retina and are seen best.

Myopia commonly originates in youth as the eye grows. Typically, a grade school or high school student experiences difficulty in reading the blackboard from far, or in seeing a movie from the rear of the theater. The condition persists throughout life. Myopes always will require glasses (or contact lenses) to see distant objects clearly.

Hyperopia may be congenital. **Presbyopia** commonly arises and progresses from ages 45–60. Presby-

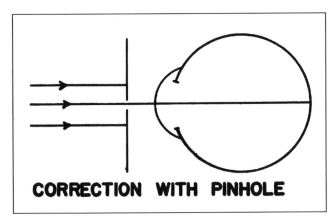

Figure 9-35

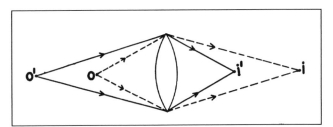

Figure 9-37

opes have difficulty seeing near objects clearly, as do hyperopes, but the mechanism is different. The lens becomes less resilient with age and does not thicken as readily on accommodation; hence, the accommodative effort is less effective in presbyopia and near vision is poor. At first the patient may try to compensate for the low lens resiliency by trying very hard to accommodate, supercontracting the ciliary muscles. He may even be successful in the effort, but at the expense of inducing headache or fatigue. He may try to compensate by holding the newspaper farther away, wishing his arms were longer. Eventually, though, reading glasses become necessary to provide the additional focusing power.

Fig. 9-38. Presbyopia.

The percentage of patients requiring glasses by age 60 in order to see perfectly for both near and far is close to 100%. The patient who never had a refractive error requires reading glasses (positive; convex lenses) for presbyopia as the eyes change between ages 45–60. The myopic patient may compensate for the need for reading glasses (plus lenses) by simply removing her myopic glasses (i.e. removes her negative, concave lenses). However, she still, and always will, require glasses to see far.

The hyperopic patient who sees far well may never require glasses for distance. At some point he will require them for near, and at an earlier age than the patient who has no refractive error.

CASE HISTORY: Sam was a smart young intern. He always carried around a small Rosenbaum near vision-testing card and routinely used it in his workups. The

Rosenbaum card, of course, is the "equivalent" of the Snellen chart. Although the patient stands 20 feet away from a Snellen chart and only 14 inches from the Rosenbaum card, the letters are proportionally smaller on the Rosenbaum card to compensate for the patient being closer. One day, Sam became extremely perplexed. He had a patient with a cataract. The patient had 20/100 vision (i.e. saw at 20 feet from the chart what a person with normal vision would see at 100 feet from the chart) in the affected eye, whether using the Snellen chart or the Rosenbaum card. There was nothing unexpected about this; the near and far charts were "equivalent." Sam noticed, however, that his own vision (without glasses) was 20/100 for far (the Snellen chart), but an excellent 20/20 for near (the Rosenbaum card). "Something must be wrong with these charts," Sam thought. "I used good illumination and was the proper distance from the charts. I should have equal vision with either chart because the charts are 'equivalent'." Sam consulted with his attending physician, who was not especially noted for keen judgment or knowledge. The attending tried the charts himself and, to his surprise, found that without his glasses he saw perfectly well for far but saw 20/100 for near. "Obviously", the attending commented "these charts work only on patients." How does one account for these discrepancies?

ANS: Fig. 9-39 illustrates why the Snellen and Rosenbaum charts are "equivalent."

Fig. 9-39 The basis for equivalency of the near and far vision charts. In order to see clearly, an image must not only be sharply focused on the retina but must be large enough. A microscopic object cannot be seen even when sharply focused. Patients may thus improve poor vision

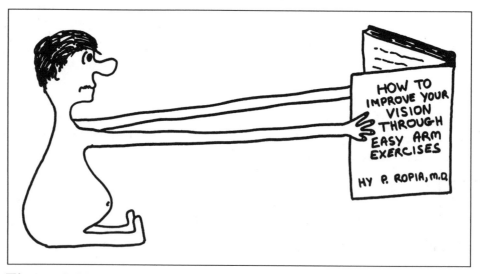

Figure 9-38

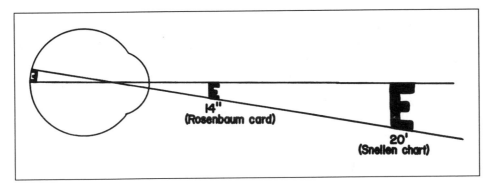

Figure 9-39

by using a magnifying glass. The Rosenbaum and Snellen charts are "equivalent" only in that they both project the same sized images on the retina. If order to clearly see the letters, however, the eyes must focus them. The attending was presbyopic and had difficulty focusing for near. Sam was myopic. He saw perfectly for near but could not focus for far. Both Sam and the attending had refractive errors. The patient had a non-refractive problem; focusing worked fine for the patient. The patient's problem was one of the cloudiness of the lens. One would expect his vision to be as poor for near as for far.

QUESTION: Which method should the physician use for routine visual testing, the near chart or distant chart?

ANS: If one wishes to be certain that a patient has no difficulty in visual acuity, both near and far must be tested. Certainly, testing far vision alone is insufficient for the middle age patient who reports headaches, fatigue and blurred vision on reading up close. Near testing must be performed to evaluate for presbyopia. Similarly, when a teenager reports difficulty seeing distant objects, near vision testing is insufficient. Sometimes, the physician is selectively interested in determining whether the patient has a non-refractive error (e.g., visual loss from acute ocular trauma). Under such conditions it may suffice to test either near or far vision as the finding of normal vision for either would rule out visual loss from such a condition. In general, it is best to test both near and far vision.

Astigmatism

A spherical lens bends light equally all around its circumference. A cylindrical lens bends light only along one axis, as only one of its axes is curved.

Fig. 9-40. Refraction through a spherical and a cylindrical lens. A spherical refractive error is erased by introducing a spherical lens of opposite refractive

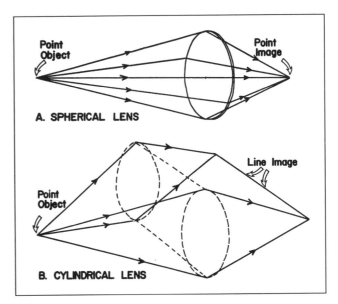

Figure 9-40

properties. A cylindrical refractive error (**astigmatism**) is corrected by introducing a cylindrical lens of opposite refractive properties. Patients may have a combination of astigmatism and a spherical refractive error. In that case the physician may correct the problem by combining a spherical lens with a cylindrical lens placed along the appropriate axis.

Reading Prescriptions

The following is a sample eyeglass prescription:

OD −2.00 +0.75 × 180
OS −1.75 +0.25 × 180 Add +1.50 ou

This means: In the right eye (OD) the correction calls for a minus (concave) 2.00 diopter spherical lens, combined with a plus (convex) 0.75 cylindrical lens that is placed at an axis of 180°. The left eye requires a minus 1.75 spherical lens combined with a +0.25 cylinder at 180°. In addition, the patient has difficulty with near vision (probably presbyopia) and requires for each eye (ou) a plus 1.50 spherical lens added on to the rest of the prescription as a bifocal segment, for near vision. The bifocal add is generally placed at the bottom of the eyeglasses as it is used when the patient is looking down to focus on near objects, particularly in reading.

Amblyopia and Strabismus

Amblyopia is a visual loss with no apparent gross pathology. There is no cloudiness of the cornea or lens, or apparent retinal lesions. Amblyopia is not corrected by glasses. It is a microscopic defect in the wiring of the retina-to-brain connections that results from disuse of one eye at an early age (generally before age 7). An adult who does not use an eye will not develop amblyopia. A child below age 7 who does not use an eye will develop amblyopia, and the condition may become irreversible if not corrected quickly. Amblyopia occurs in only one eye. It is proposed that connections in the brain from one eye do not develop well if that eye is not used. Instead, connection sites are usurped by nerve fibers from the good eye. After maturity, correcting the cause of amblyopia will not restore function, as the connection (synaptic) sites are already filled by permanent connections from the normal eye.

There are three main causes of amblyopia—physical occlusion (as by cataract or ptosis), refractive errors, and strabismus. **Strabismus**, which affects about 2–3% of the population, is an abnormal turning of the eye either inward (crossed eyes; **esotropia**) or outward (walleyes; **exotropia**). If a child's eye has a refractive error, in effect that eye suffers from disuse and develops amblyopia. The treatment for refractive amblyopia is early correction of visual acuity.

Amblyopia caused by strabismus is also the product of disuse. A child with crossed eyes does not see double. Rather, she learns to suppress the vision in one eye to avoid seeing double. The suppressed eye, in effect, experiences "disuse" and becomes amblyopic. The initial treatment for strabismic amblyopia is to force the use of the eye by covering the normal eye. Correction of the strabismus is also part of the treatment. This sometimes requires surgery. At other times, particularly when the basis for strabismus is an overconvergence of the eyes on attempted accommodation (the eyes normally converge when accommodating), treatment may be accomplished by accommodating for the patient without demanding extraocular muscle movement. That is, glasses, or special eye drops (e.g. phospholine iodide, a long-acting anticholinesterase) that constrict the ciliary muscles, are sometimes employed effectively. An adult who develops strabismus (e.g. from trauma) does not suppress vision in one eye, but sees double for the rest of his life.

When children with amblyopia wear a patch over the good eye, the eye with poor vision is forced into seeing and may improve. Surgery for strabismus generally has better results when both eyes see well. It important to alternate the patch from one eye to the other, as amblyopia may be induced in the good eye by covering it for too many days!

Color Vision

Defective color vision is a hereditary condition based on a defective recessive gene on the X chromosome. Therefore, it is far more common in males than in females, affecting about 6% of males and 0.6% of females.

There are two types of photoreceptors in the retina—rods and cones. The cones are especially clustered in the foveal area of the retina, the region in the center of the retina with the greatest visual acuity. A key reason for the the high visual acuity of cones is their almost one-to-one connection with bipolar cells and ganglion cells. The rods lie more peripherally. Thousands of rods may converge on a single ganglion cell, and the rods therefore have poorer visual acuity than the cones, but they are more sensitive to dim light.

Unlike the rods, the cones perceive color. There are three types of cone color photoreceptors in the retina—red, green and blue, which together operate to perceive the colors of the spectrum (see Fig. 9-6). Color blindness may result from deficits in any of these kinds of cones. Most color blind individuals have difficulty distinguishing reds and greens. Rarely, the defect may involve difficulty distinguishing blues and yellows. Various color plate charts (e.g. the Ishihara or American Optical color plates) are used to detect these deficiences. The tests consists of pictures of letters or numbers composed of various colored dots. Incorrect perception of the figures occurs with defective color vision.

THE SPECIAL SENSES: HEARING

Fig. 9-41. The auditory system. An explorer crawling into the external acoustic meatus would reach a dead end at the ear drum (**tympanic membrane**), which marks the transition from outer to middle ear. The eardrum is tilted as as if it would fall on top of the explorer. The drum is cone-shaped, seemingly prevented from falling by its attachment to the chain of 3 small bones (ossicles) of the middle ear cavity.

These bones are:

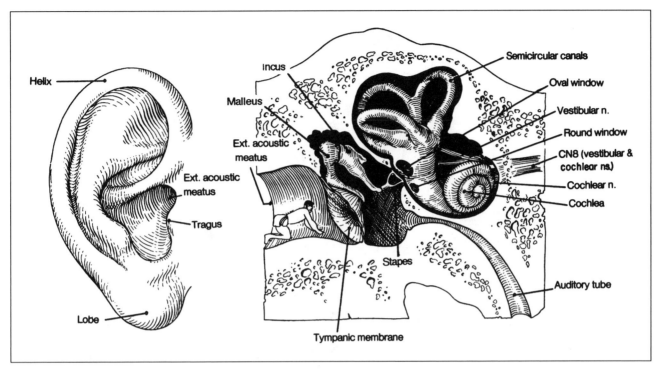

Figure 9-41

1) The **malleus** (hammer), which attaches directly to the drum by its handle.
2) The **incus** (anvil)
3) The **stapes** (stirrup)

The three ear bones vibrate rapidly and relay sound impulses from the tympanic membrane to the oval window. The oval window is a hole in the bone that marks the transition from middle ear to inner ear. The stapes attaches to the oval window, behaving like a nervous door knocker that vibrates very rapidly. Actually, the 3 bones look like a muscle-man standing on top of the tympanic membrane and about to swat the explorer with a tennis racquet. Fortunately, the tennis racquet is stuck to the oval window.

Fig. 9-42. The inner ear. The explorer could leave the middle ear by sliding down the auditory (Eustachian) tube in the anteroinferior aspect of the middle ear or by climbing up into a hole in the roof, the mastoid antrum. The explorer opts, instead, to go scuba diving. Rather than leave through air-filled passages, he dons a scuba outfit, cuts out the stapes, enters the oval window, and swims into the inner ear, specifically into the perilymph of the vestibule.

Normally, the inner ear (cochlea) is rolled up like a snail shell. It is here schematically unrolled as if some-one blew out a New Year's Eve noisemaker. The scala vestibuli gets it name from the fact that it connects directly with the vestibule, or entrance, to the inner ear. The **PERIlymph** gets its name from the fact that it occupies the outer, or more peripheral of the two fluid-filled chambers (the other chamber contains **ENDOlymph**).

Sound waves passing across the oval window travel in the **scala vestibuli** and are transmitted to the **cochlear duct** where they vibrate the **tectorial membrane**, stimulating specialized receptor cells in the **organ of Corti** (Fig. 9-43). The specialized receptor cells at each point along the length of the tectorial membrane respond to a different frequency of fluid vibration, thereby enabling the person to distinguish different pitches. Whereas pitch is determined by frequency of vibration, loudness is determined by amplitude of vibration.

Fig. 9-43. Cross section through: A. A semicircular canal, B. The cochlea. Both have a "balloon-within-a balloon" pattern.

(1) semicircular canal (contains perilymph as do the scala vestibuli and scala tympani)
(2) semicircular duct (endolymph)
(3) vestibular membrane (angled, like the side of a "V")

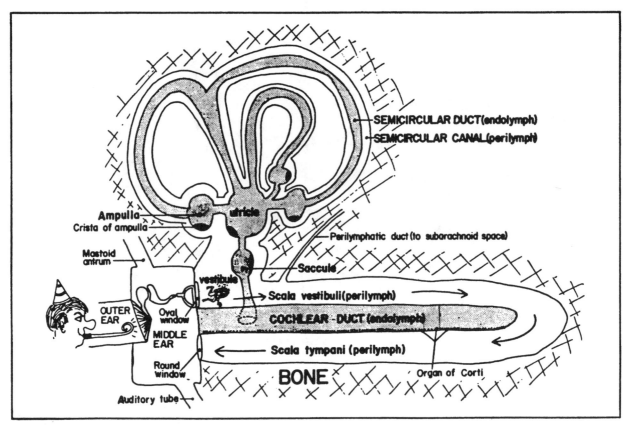

Figure 9-42

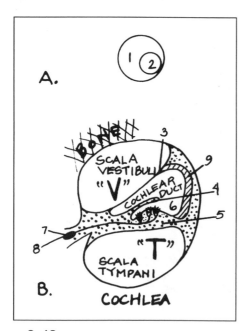

Figure 9-43

(4) tectorial membrane (moves and stimulates neurosensitive hair cells of the organ of Corti)
(5) scala Tympani (its top runs straight across, like the top of a "T")
(6) organ of Corti
(7) spiral ganglion
(8) cochlear nerve
(9) vascular stria (produces endolymph)

Impulses from the organ of Corti travel along cochlear nerve fibers, in company with vestibular nerve fibers from the saccule, utricle and semicircular canals, to the brain stem.

The three **semicircular canals** are shaped somewhat like a pretzel. These three canals lie at right angles to one another. Their three **ampullae** contain neurosensitive structures (**cristae**) that respond to differential fluid movement in the canals and can sense sudden rotational movements of the head.

The saccule and utricle each contain a **macula** ("sac" rhymes with "mac"), a motion-sensitive structure which is covered by a gelatinous substance that contains calcium carbonate crystals (**statoconia**, or **otoliths**). Sensitive hair cells in the macula protrude in all directions. Movements of the crystals in relation to head movements or gravity stimulate the sensory receptors and help determine the position of the head, whether in static conditions or in motion.

If the diver continues swimming in the perilymph, he will reach the scala tympani, a continuation of the perilymph that will carry the diver full circle back toward the tympanic cavity (middle ear). The diver will not enter the middle ear because the round window obstructs the way. The round window has no ossicles attached to it and thus is not distorted out of shape like the oval window. Piercing through the round window, the explorer would reenter the middle ear. If the explorer

wished, he could have entered the subarachnoid space of the brain via the **perilymphatic duct** or swum around in the perilymph of the utricle, saccule, and semicircular canals. He would not, however, have swum in any endolymph, which occupies a separate internal chamber (the balloon within a balloon). The endolymph, like the perilymph, may be found in the cochlea (specifically in the cochlear duct) as well as in the saccule, utricle, and semicircular ducts. The endolymph fluid has a different chemical composition than the perilymph.

The explorer was wise in leaving through the round window, rather than exploring the vestibular system for that would take him through a SEWER system (SUA= Saccule, Utricle, and Ampulla of the semicircular canals).

CHAPTER 10.   THE DIGESTIVE SYSTEM

Efficient food intake requires gastrointestinal **motility**, **digestion** and **absorption**. Malfunction may occur in any of the above categories.

Motility

After the teeth chew the food, thereby providing greater surface area for digestion, swallowing occurs through the combined action of the tongue and pharyngeal muscles. The upper third of the esophagus is under voluntary control, whereas the musculature in the lower portion becomes progressively more involuntary.

Throughout the gastrointestinal (GI) tract, there is a pattern of musculature characterized by a combination of circular and longitudinal muscle at any given point (Fig. 10-1). This arrangement allows the food to be pushed along (**peristalsis**) in addition to being mixed. After swallowing, it takes about 1-3 hours for solid food to leave the stomach and about 4-6 hours beyond that to reach the ileocecal valve. Typically, it takes about 1-2 days for food to completely pass through the digestive system.

The vagus nerve functions as a fine tuner of digestion. It stimulates peristaltic movements, usually relaxes digestive sphincters, and also promotes GI secretion. As one might expect, the vagal nerve fibers that influence motility (**myenteric plexus**) are located strategically between the circular and longitudinal muscle layers, whereas those that influence secretion (**Meissner's plexus**) lie near the glandular regions in the submucosa. The same is true of the sympathetic system, which has effects opposite to that of the parasympathetics.

Fig. 10-1.   Schematic view of a cross section through the GI tract.

Digestion and Absorption

Among the numerous digestion-related molecules, some directly attack and digest the food, whereas others have cell-regulatory effects. For instance, amylases, pepsin, maltase, lactase, sucrase, peptidases, lipases, trypsin, chymotrypsin, procarboxypolypeptidase, cholesterol esterase, phospholipase and nucleases digest food. Histamine, gastrin, secretin, gastric inhibitory peptide, cholecystokinin, pancreozymin and enterokinase participate in digestion by interacting with other cells or enzymes. Some molecules act locally (e.g. intestinal peptidases digest food in the intestine), while others circulate as hormones (e.g. gastrin, secretin, gastric inhibitory peptide, cholecystokinin, pancreozymin).

Fig. 10-2.   Digestive chemicals. The body's energy comes from carbohydrates, fats, and proteins, which must be broken down to readily absorbed forms. Fat provides the most energy per gram (carbohydrates 4.0 Cal/gm; protein 4.0 Cal/gm; fat 9.0 Cal/gm). In starvation, carbohydrate is depleted within a day; then, for the most part, fat is used, and finally protein.

The splitting of complex carbohydrates, proteins and fats involves hydrolysis (the addition of water during the splitting process). This may occur partially at first, but is completed in the small intestine. In general, molecules secreted at a particular level of the digestive system act at that level to promote digestion, whereas they may feed back negatively to inhibit digestion at a preceeding point of the digestive tract. For instance, the hormone cholecystokinin which is released from the small intestine, stimulates pancreatic enzyme secretion and gall bladder contraction, but decreases gastric motility. Gastrin, produced in the stomach, enhances gastric secretion of HCl and pepsinogen and enhances stomach contraction. Secretin and gastric inhibitory peptide (GIP), hormones secreted in the small intestine, decrease gastrin secretion.

Negative feedback occurs via the nervous system, too; digestive products may influence digestion by stimulating local reflex arcs that are confined to the GI tract. For example, excess distension of the duodenum with chyme stimulates a local reflex within the myenteric plexus that decreases gastric motility and emptying. Or, messages may spread back to the central nervous system via the autonomic nervous system, which will then respond by fine-tuning digestion.

Insulin and glucagon, while not thought of customarily as digestion-related hormones, do have some effect on intestinal motility. Insulin increases and glucagon decreases intestinal motility. Glucagon may be given intravenously during a barium enema x-ray to reduce colon motility and decrease the patient's discomfort during the procedure.

Fig. 10-3.   Digestion of carbohydrates. Starches (e.g. amylose; glycogen) are polymers of glucose ($C_6H_{12}O_6$). Maltose, lactose and sucrose are disaccharides (Maltose = glucose + glucose; Lactose = glucose + galactose; Sucrose = glucose + fructose). Absorption of carbohydrates requires that they first be broken down to monosaccharides, namely glucose, galactose, and fructose, which are then absorbed into the small intestine, where they enter the portal blood. This occurs partly through enzymes released by the salivary, intestinal and pancreatic glands. HCl in the stomach also has a small effect in the hydrolysis of starches.

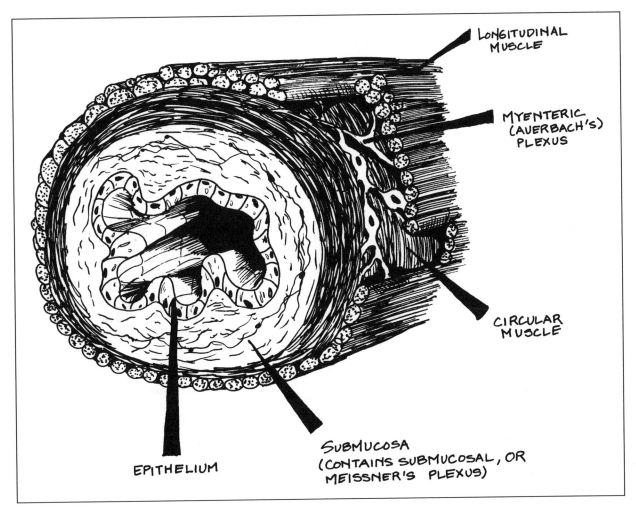

Figure 10-1

Proteins need to be broken down to amino acids, but small peptides can also be absorbed (one of the causes of allergies to certain proteins). Protein digestion begins in the stomach with HCl and pepsin, and ends in the small intestine with trypsin, chymotrypsin, and carboxypolypeptidase from the pancreas, and intestinal peptidases.

Fig. 10-4. Fat digestion. **Lipids** (fats) must be split by a variety of lipase enzymes. Fat leaving the stomach is first emulsified (broken into small droplets), partly through the gastrointestinal churning process and partly through the influence of bile salts. The emulsion drops provide a broad surface area on which lipid digestion can occur. Pancreatic and intestinal lipases break down triglycerides to monoglycerides and free fatty acids. Pancreatic and intestinal esterases break down cholesterol esters to free cholesterol and free fatty acids. Pancreatic phospholipases remove fatty acids from phospholipids, leaving lysophospholipids (phospholipids missing a fatty acid molecule) and free fatty acids.

The bile sale molecules then mix with the free fatty acids, monoglycerides, cholesterol and lysophospholipids to form **micelles**, tiny carrier vehicles (much small than the emulsion drops) that transport the digested lipid products to the brush borders of intestinal epithelial cells for absorption.

The fact that bile salt molecules have a polar end (which points outward to the aqueous **chyme**, chyme being a euphemism for vomit) and a non-polar end (which points inward) enables the micelles to be soluble in chyme in addition to solubilizing and transporting the relatively polar lipids.

Inside the intestinal epithelial cell, the free fatty acids recombine with the monoglycerides, free cholesterol and lysophospholipids to form, respectively, triglycerides, cholesterol esters and phospholipids. These, together with **apoproteins** (proteins that become active when combined with something else) form **chylomicrons**, which are extruded from the cell to en-

ORGAN/CELL TYPE	CHEMICAL PRODUCED	FUNCTION
MOUTH		
Salivary Glands	Mucus	Lubricant
	Salivary Amylase	Partially breaks down starch to maltose, maltotriose, and alpha limit dextrins
	Antibodies and proteolytic enzymes	Antibiotic effect
ESOPHAGUS		
Mucous Cell	Mucus	Lubricant
STOMACH		
Chief Cell (= peptic cell) (Stimulated by gastrin, pepsin, and HCL)	Pepsinogen	Changes to pepsin in presence of H^+ to break down proteins to peptides.
Parietal Cell (= oxyntic cell) (Stimulated by vagus, gastrin, histamine, amino acids and peptides in stomach and duodenum. Stimulated by local and central reflexes from gastric and duodenal distention. Inhibited by low gastric and intestinal pH, and fat in intestinal chyme, via secretin, cholecystokinin, GIP, somatostatin secretion and local neural relexes.)	HCl	Facilitates pepsinogen change to pepsin; mild hydrolysis of starches; bacterocidal; pH facilitates some mineral absorption in intestine (e.g. iron).
	Intrinsic Factor	Binds to B12 and facilitates its absorption in small intestine.
Mucous Neck Cell	Mucus	Protects mucosa from acid and pepsin
Surface epithelial cells	Bicarbonate	Protects mucosa against acid.
Mucosal Cells in Gastric Antrum	Histamine	Diffuses to stimulate parietal cells to produce acid, in conjunction with gastrin and vagal acetylcholine.
Gastrin Cells in Antrum (Stimulated by vagus, by distension of duodenum, and by peptides; Inhibited by secretin, GIP and excess acidity)	Gastrin	Via blood stream, stimulates parietal cells to secrete HCl; Increases intestinal motility; stimulates pyloric contraction and relaxation of pyloric sphincter; stimulates pancreatic enzyme secretion; relaxes ileocecal valve.

Figure 10-2 (continued)

ORGAN/CELL TYPE	CHEMICAL PRODUCED	FUNCTION
DUODENUM/SMALL INTESTINE		
Brunners's glands	alkaline mucus	Protects duodenum from stomach acidity.
Epithelial cells of Crypts of Lieberkuhn in intestinal villi (Vagus stimulates secretion in general; digestive enzyme secretion is stimulated by direct contact with food. Fat and acid stimulate secretin, GIP, and cholecystokinin secretion.)	Mucus	Lubricant, protective
	Maltase	Splits maltose to 2 glucose units
	Lactase	Splits lactose to glucose and galactose
	Sucrase	Splits sucrose to glucose and fructose.
	Peptidases	Break down small peptides to amino acids.
	Intestinal Lipase	Breaks down fats to glycerol and fatty acids
	Intestinal esterases	Break down cholesterol esters to free cholesterol and fatty acids.
	Secretin	Decreases gastrin secretion and motility; stimulates bile sale secretion in liver and pancreatic bicarbonate secretion; inhibits gastrointestinal motility.
	Gastric inhibitory peptide (GIP)	Inhibits gastrin secretion; decreases the speed of gastric emptying
	Cholecystokinin	Decreases gastric motility; stimulates pancreatic enzyme and bicarbonate secretion; stimulates gall bladder contraction and relaxation of sphincter of Oddi; causes vasodilation in intestinal mucosa.
	Enterokinase	Activates changes of trypsinogen to trypsin; chymotrypsinogen to chymotrypsin; procarboxypolypeptidase to carboxypolypeptidase.
	Bulbogastrone	Inhibits parietal cell acid secretion.
PANCREAS (EXOCRINE)		
Pancreatic ductule cells	Bicarbonate	Neutralizes stomach acid
Exocrine cells (Secretion stimulated by vagus, cholecysto-kinin, and secretin)	Pancreatic Amylase	Changes starch to oligosaccharides.
	Trypsinogen (activated by enterokinase)	Break down proteins to peptides and amino acids.

Figure 10-2 (continued)

ORGAN/CELL TYPE	CHEMICAL PRODUCED	FUNCTION
	Chymotrypsinogen (activated by trypsin)	
	Procarboxypolypeptidase (activated by trypsin)	
	Pancreatic Lipase	Breaks down triglycerides to fatty acids and monoglycerides
	Cholesterol Esterase	Cleaves cholesterol esters to free cholesterol and fatty acids.
	Phospholipase	Removes fatty acids from phospholipids.
	Nucleases	Change nucleic acids to nucleotides
(ENDOCRINE)		
Beta islet cells	Insulin	Increases intestinal motility
Alpha islet cells	Glucagon	Decreases intestinal motility
Delta islet cells	Somatostatin	General effects in decreasing digestion and absorption; inhibits insulin and glucagon secretion.
LIVER **Liver cells**	Bile salts	Bile salt micelles emulsify fats into smaller particles that can be attacked by pancreatic lipase. Micelles carry fats to villi for absorption. Bile salt excretion decreases body cholesterol.
GALL BLADDER (Contraction stimulated by choecystokinin; inhibited by vagus)		Bile storage
COLON (**Mucous and epithelial cells** stimulated by vagus and by direct contact with food; inhibited by sympathetics)	Mucus	Lubrication, protection, solidifies feces.
	Bicarbonate	Helps neutralize bacterial products.

Figure 10-2 (concluded)

ter the lymphatics. Short-chain fatty acids, being relatively water soluble, can reach the liver via the portal vein. Absorbed carbohydrates and amino acids also enter the portal blood.

Fig. 10-5. The structure of lipoprotein trams, including chylomicrons, VLDL (very low density lipoproteins), LDL (low density lipoproteins), and HDL (high density lipoproteins).

Fig. 10-6. The distribution of lipoproteins in the body. Chylomicrons form in the intestinal epithelial cells that absorb the digested fats. Other lipoprotein vehicles (VLDL, LDL, IDL, HDL) form after further processing in the liver. Cholesterol is found in all lipoprotein vehicles but is relatively concentrated in LDL and HDL, whereas triglycerides are relatively concentrated in chylomicrons and VLDL. The chylomicrons drop off their triglycerides largely in fat, skeletal, and heart muscles

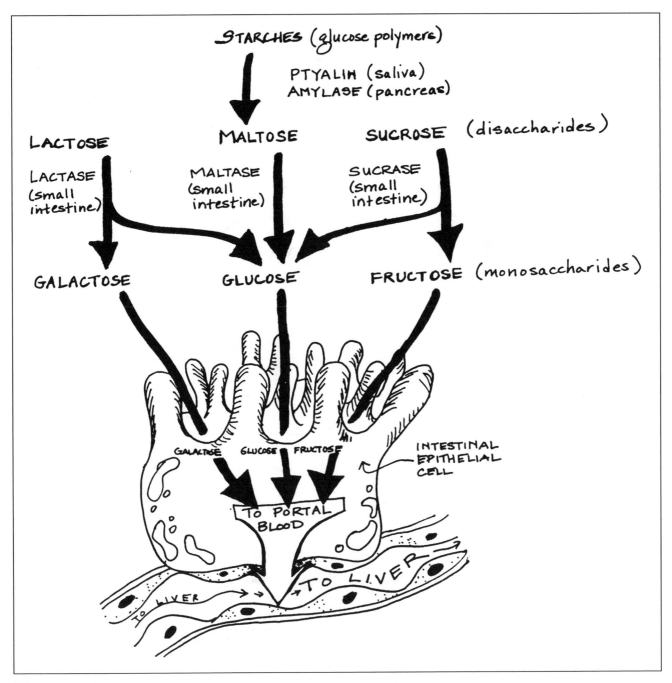

Figure 10-3

cells. A separate lipoprotein lipase, on the capillary endothelial cells of the muscle and fat tissues, first releases free fatty acids from the triglycerides. The free fatty acids then enter the muscle or fat cells, where they may be reesterified to triglycerides. That's a lot of work, but then again, fatty acids are used as energy sources.

Absorption of fat is completed by the end of the jejunum, but reabsorption of the bile salts occurs in the ileum in what is termed the **enterohepatic circulation**, a recycling of bile salts from intestine to portal blood to liver to bile ducts to intestine.

Absorption of fatty acids and monoglycerides appears to be passive, via simple diffusion. Much of the absorption of amino acids, carbohydrates, calcium, iron, other minerals, and some of the vitamins is facilitated by a secondary active cotransport mechanism with sodium, sim-

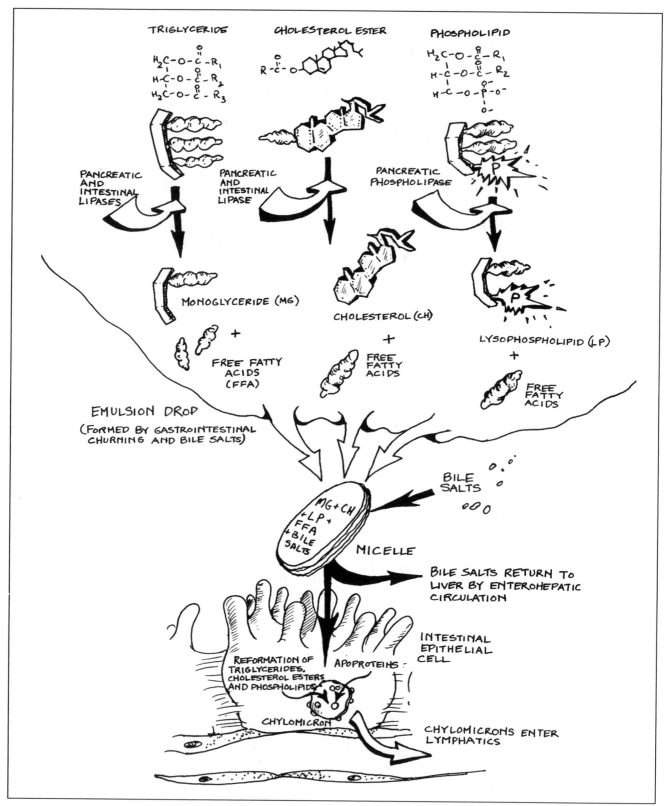

Figure 10-4

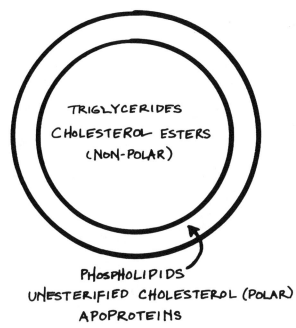

TRIGLYCERIDES
CHOLESTEROL ESTERS
(NON-POLAR)

PHOSPHOLIPIDS
UNESTERIFIED CHOLESTEROL (POLAR)
APOPROTEINS

Figure 10-5

ilar to that in the renal tubule (Fig. 1-3). The process is driven by a sodium/potassium ATPase pump. Water absorption follows passively and is most prominent in the small intestine, a lesser amount occurring in the colon.

When Things Go Wrong

Digestive difficulties include disorders of motility, digestion and absorption.

In **achalasia** there is a defect in esophageal smooth muscle motility and in relaxation of the lower esophageal sphincter. The patient can swallow, but food is held up from passing to the stomach. There is believed to be a defect in the myenteric neurons. In **Hirschsprung's megacolon,** there is a similar defect, but in the colon, resulting in poor colonic motility and a dilated colon.

Far more common manifestations of abnormal motility are constipation and diarrhea. It should be noted, though, that diarrhea is not necessarily due to increased bowel motility, but may also be due to increased secretions from intestinal irritation. One of the worst forms of diarrhea occurs with **cholera** toxin. This causes marked secretion of Cl- in the intestinal lumen, with water passively following the chloride.

Malabsorption of food may occur either with inadequate digestion or with inadequate absorption of adequately digested food. In **lactose intolerance,** for

instance, there is a deficiency of lactase, leading to cramping abdominal pain and diarrhea. There is **vitamin B12 deficiency** in **pernicious anemia,** an autoimmune disease that affects the gastric mucosa. The mucosal damage causes a deficiency in secretion of **intrinsic factor,** which is necessary for B12 absorption. There commonly is also a decrease in stomach acidity (**achlorhydria**) since the same cells (gastric parietal cells) that secrete intrinsic factor also secrete HCl.

In **celiac disease,** the intestinal villi are damaged by sensitivity to gluten, which is found in wheat and rye. In that case, food, although adequately digested, is not adequately absorbed. It may first come to attention through the appearance of fatty stools (**steatorrhea**), but may lead to multiple nutritional deficiencies. Malabsorption of fat will also result in malabsorption of fat-soluble vitamins (D,E,A, and K).

Clinical problems may also result from excess secretion. Duodenal ulcers commonly are associated with excess gastric acidity. Ulcers may also result from inadequate mucus production or decreased alkaline pancreatic secretion. (Actually gastric ulcers are commonly associated with **decreased** acid production, and may result from defects in factors that normally protect the gastric mucosa.) In the **Zollinger-Ellison syndrome** severe duodenal ulceration results from gastrin-producing tumors that induce marked gastric acidity. H2 blockers (e.g. cimetidine), which block histamine receptors, may be used to decrease acid production in duodenal ulcer disease. In **pancreatitis** there is premature activation of pancreatic enzymes, which then damage the pancreas. **Gall stone** precipitation may result from an excess in the normal cholesterol/bile salt ratio.

The Vitamins

Vitamins are chemicals that are necessary in trace amounts for normal body function. They are not produced in sufficient amounts by the body and must come from external food sources. Their structures are generally diverse and unrelated, as shown in Figs. 10-7 and 10-8.

It is useful to divide vitamins into water soluble and fat-soluble groups:

Fig. 10-7. The water-soluble vitamins.

Fig. 10-8. The fat-soluble vitamins.

Water-soluble vitamins (B1, B2, B6, B12, C, folacin, biotin, niacin, pantothenate) generally wash out of foods easily, and also wash out of the body relatively easily, (hence, are less easily stored in the body—an exception is vitamin B12 which is stored excellently, particularly in the liver). One may thus become depleted relatively quickly of most water soluble vitamins. Fortunately, so

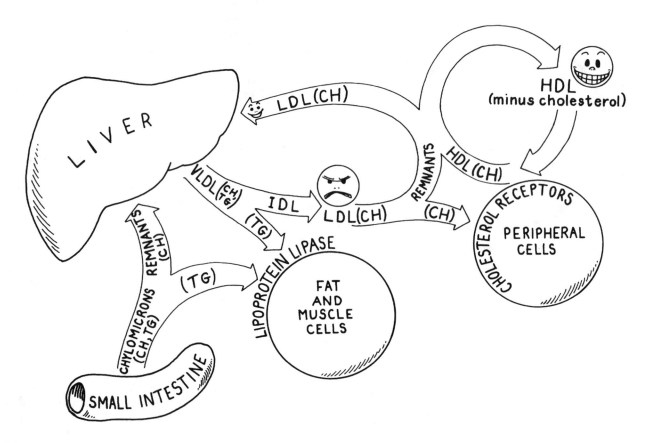

Figure 10-6

many foods are rich in them. Toxicity reactions, on the other hand, are more likely with fat-soluble vitamins, as they are so well-stored and are not eliminated easily from the body.

Deficiency of any of the vitamins may occur with inadequate intake. Fat-soluble vitamin deficiency may particularly occur in clinical conditions that affect fat absorption in the gut. Other intestinal wall diseases may affect vitamin absorption in general, causing deficiency of both water and fat soluble vitamins.

Vitamin D is partly produced by the skin on exposure to sunlight; vitamin K and biotin are produced in part by intestinal bacteria; and vitamin B12 is especially well-stored. Hence, it is uncommon to have a deficiency of these vitamins on the basis of dietary intake alone. Infants, who have less bacterial intestinal flora and relatively little stores of vitamin K have a greater need than adults for vitamin K in the diet.

Clinical points relevant to specific water-soluble vitamins are as follows:

VITAMIN B1 (thiamine):
COMMON FOOD SOURCES: wheat germ and whole grain cereals; fish, meat, eggs, milk, green vegetables
DEFICIENCY RESULTS IN: 1) **Beri-beri**. This is associated with a diet of refined rice or with excess cooking of food, which decreases B1 through washing out or through heating. The patient experiences cardiac and neurologic complications such as palpitations, edema, general weakness, pins-and-needles sensations and pain in the legs. 2) **Wernicke-Korsakoff syndrome**. This is correlated with alcoholism, but appears to be due to a nutritional deficiency rather than direct effects of alcohol. It may exist as a separate hereditary condition requiring large amounts of thiamine. There is a psychosis, with confabulation (fabrication of stories) and recent memory loss and other neurologic problems (nystagmus, eye muscle weakness, poor muscle coordination). Alcoholics undergoing delirium tremens (DTs) commonly receive intravenous thiamine as part of their in-hospital therapy

VITAMIN B2 (Riboflavin):

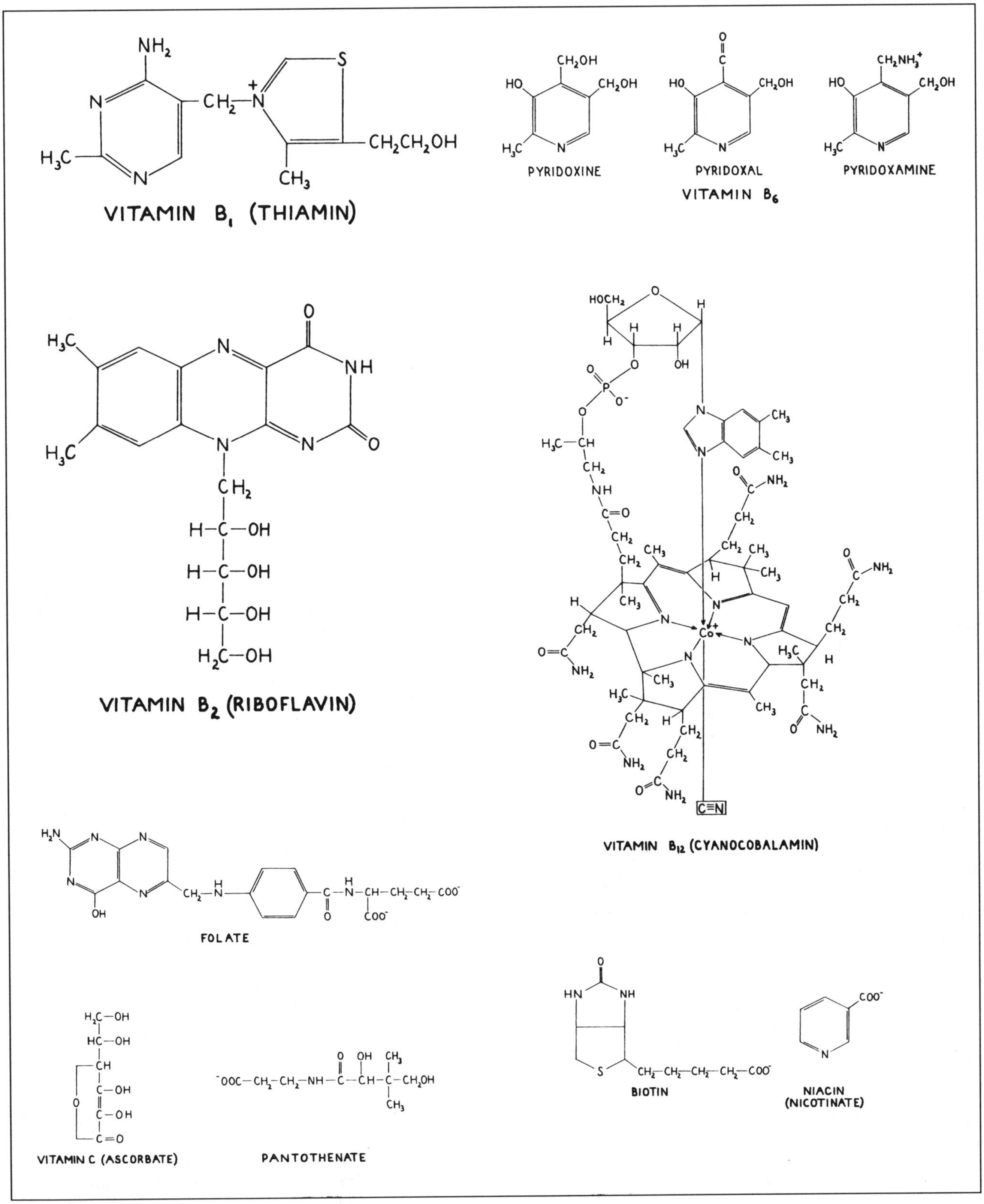
VITAMIN B1 (THIAMIN)
PYRIDOXINE
PYRIDOXAL
PYRIDOXAMINE
VITAMIN B6
VITAMIN B2 (RIBOFLAVIN)
VITAMIN B12 (CYANOCOBALAMIN)
FOLATE
BIOTIN
NIACIN
(NICOTINATE)
VITAMIN C (ASCORBATE)
PANTOTHENATE

Figure 10-7

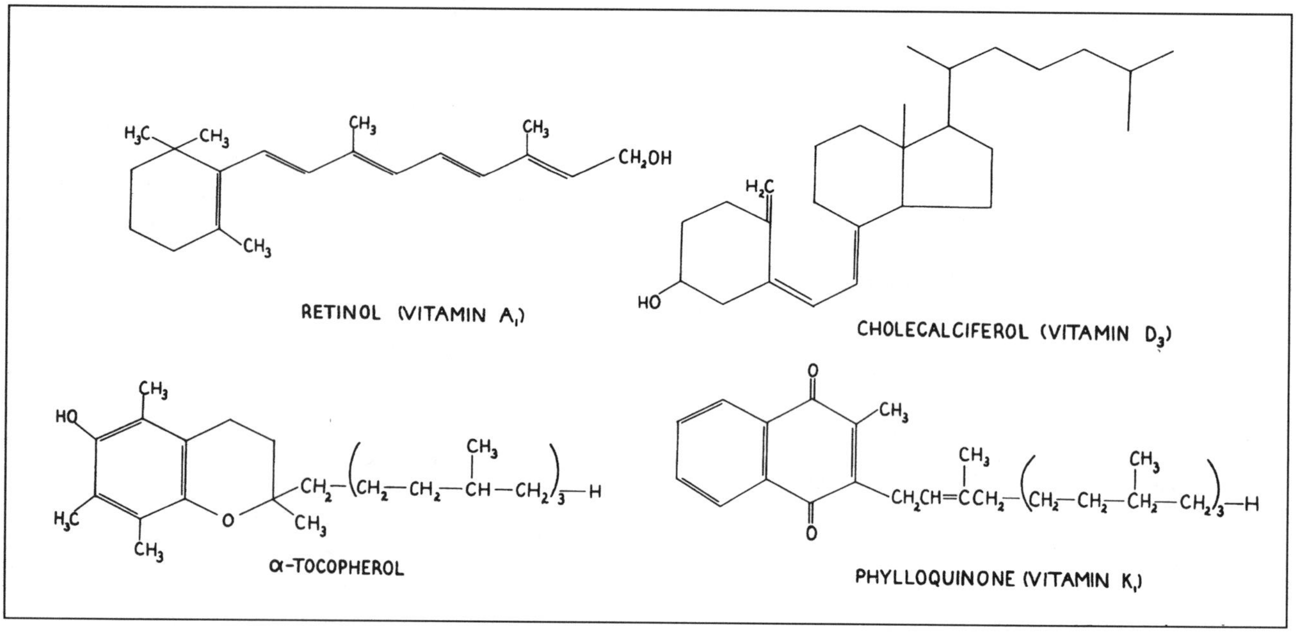

Figure 10-8

COMMON FOOD SOURCES: fish, meat, eggs, milk, green vegetables.

DEFICIENCY RESULTS IN: angular stomatitis (cracks in the corner of the mouth), inflammation of the tongue, seborrheic dermatitis, and anemia.

VITAMIN B6 (pyridoxin; pyridoxal; pyrodoxamine):

COMMON FOOD SOURCES: whole grain cereals, fish, meat, eggs, green vegetables.

DEFICIENCY RESULTS IN: dermatitis, glossitis, anemia, and neurologic disturbances such as peripheral neuropathy and convulsions.

COMMENT: Deficiency is rare, as B6 is so common in foods. Isoniazid, an antituberculosis drug, can interfere with B6 and induce symptoms of B6 deficiency. As pyridoxine is necessary in the steps that convert tryptophan to niacin, a deficiency of B6 may result in niacin deficiency.

VITAMIN B12 (cyanocobolamin):

COMMON FOOD SOURCES: Only microorganisms make B12 (not even plants make it). Large quantities are stored in the body, especially in the liver, enough to last 3 or more years, which is not the case for other water-soluble vitamins. We acquire vitamin B12 through ingestion of meats (especially liver) and dairy products, including food fermented by bacteria, such as yogurt, soya sauce and sauerkraut.

DEFICIENCY: **Pernicious anemia.** Conceivably, one coud get B12 deficiency on a purely vegetarian diet, but this is rare. Deficiency is more likely with diseases of the intestine that impede absorption (e.g. tropical sprue, regional enteritis). The tapeworm Diphyllobothrium latum may deplete B12 stores. A deficiency of gastric intrinsic factor (a glycoprotein) may result in B12 deficiency, as intrinsic factor is important in facilitating B12 absorption in the bowel. Intrinsic factor deficiency may occur following gastrectomy or as an entity in itself, in pernicious anemia. Intrinsic factor deficiency sometimes results from an autoimmune disease.

Patients with pernicious anemia have a macrocytic anemia, hypersegmented leukocytes, and neurosensory deficits (especially poor position sense) related to degeneration of the posterior columns of the spinal cord. Diagnostic clues include decreased B12 levels in the serum; a positive Schilling test in which radioactive labeled B12 is ingested, with subsequent assays of the degree of absorption; decreased acidity of gastric secretion (as low stomach acidity is associated with lack of intrinsic factor and poor B12 absorption). Treatment of pernicious anemia consists of B12 injections to offset the poor intestinal absorption.

VITAMIN C (ascorbic acid):

COMMON FOOD SOURCES: many fruits and vegetables.

DEFICIENCY: Man, other primates, and guinea pigs cannot synthesize vitamin C. Nor is it stored in the body. Hence, the need for continued replenishment, and the development of **scurvy** with lack of vitamin C. In scurvy, there are swollen gums and easy bruisability, coinciding with defective collagen formation. Serum levels of ascorbic acid may be tested for diagnosis.

EXCESS: There is concern about the possibility that certain susceptible individuals may develop renal stones or hemolytic anemia from megadoses of vitamin C.

FOLACIN (=folate=folic acid):
COMMON FOOD SOURCES: cereals, liver, fruit, green leafy vegetables.
DEFICIENCY: Folate deficiency resembles B12 deficiency so far as the anemia goes, but without the neurologic abnormalities. Unlike B12, for which there are tremendous body stores, folate needs continued replacement, and poor diet is the most common cause of folate deficiency. Serum levels of folate may help establish the diagnosis.

BIOTIN:
COMMON FOODS: widespread in foods; also produced by intestinal bacteria.
DEFICIENCY: Deficiency of biotin is rare except in people who only eat raw eggs, as egg whites conyain **avidin**, a protein that inhibits biotin absorption. There may be a dermatitis.

NIACIN (=nicotinic acid):
COMMON FOODS: wheat germ, liver, fish, peanuts.
DEFICIENCY: **Pellagra**. Niacin may be produced from tryptophan. Niacin deficiency therefore is most likely in persons with low intake of both niacin and tryptophan. People who eat mainly corn may develop niacin deficiency, since corn is low in tryptophan. In pellagra, the patient develops the 3 **D**s: **D**iarrhea, **D**ermatitis, and **D**ementia. Diagnostic testing is difficult and may best be done by seeing improvement with niacin ingestion.

PANTHOTHENATE (=pantothenic acid):
COMMON FOODS: present in many foods.
DEFICIENCY: Deficiency is very rare. The patient experiences fatigue, nausea, vomiting, abdominal pain, and neurosensory disturbances.

Clinical conditions associated with the fat-soluble vitamins (A,D,E,K) are as follows:

VITAMIN A (retinol):
COMMON FOODS: liver, fish, fortified milk, eggs, green leafy vegetables.
DEFICIENCY: Vitamin A deficiency results in night blindness and xerophthalmia (dry cornea and conjunctiva, sometimes with ulceration of the cornea). Nonocular changes may also occur: dry skin and mucous membranes. Deficiency may result from poor dietary intake, or poor absorption, as from bowel disease, or a defect in bile flow that causes fat malabsorption. Poor protein intake may result in a reduced level of the transport protein that carries vitamin A in the blood stream.
TOXICITY: Overdosage may result in vomiting, headache, depressed mental status, hair loss, skin peeling, and sometimes death.

VITAMIN D:
COMMON FOODS: fortified milk, fish liver oils, milk products, meat.
DEFICIENCY: Deficiency causes hypocalcemia and hypophosphatemia, with resultant **rickets** (bending with poor calcification of developing bone, in children) or **osteomalacia** (decalcification and softening of bones, in adults). In both of these there is impaired mineralization. These should be distinguised from another condition, **osteoporosis**, in which there is reduction in bone mass as a whole, rather than select reduction of the mineral content.
TOXICITY: Overdosage may result in hypercalcemia and renal stones.

VITAMIN E:
COMMON FOODS: vegetable oils, green vegetables.
DEFICIENCY: Evidence is inconclusive as to what effect vitamin E deficiency may have in humans. Perhaps it may be associated with dystrophic changes in muscle, and hemolysis of red blood cells.
TOXICITY: An excess may interfere with the action of various hormones, with vitamin K and blood clotting, and with white blood cell functioning.

VITAMIN K:
COMMON FOODS: widespread in animals and plants.
DEFICIENCY: Vitamin K, among other things, is important in the blood clotting mechanism. Deficiency results in hemorrhages (especially in newborns—**hemorrhagic disease of the newborn**) and an elevated prothrombin time on laboratory testing.
TOXICITY: Hemolytic anemia; **kernicterus** (deposition of bilirubin in the brain) in newborns.
COMMENT: Dicoumarol is a drug used for its anticoagulant effect. It looks like vitamin K and interferes with its functioning in blood clotting.

CHAPTER 11. THE ENDOCRINE SYSTEM

Cytokines, in the usual context of the word, are chemicals that cells release and which influence nearby cells. When the chemical feeds back to influence the same cell that released the chemical this is an **autocrine** function. When that influence involves diffusion to nearby target cells this is a **paracrine** function. (Some cytokines, such as the interleukins, are discussed in the chapter on immunology).

Fig. 11-1. Autocrine and paracrine function.

When a secreted chemical enters the blood stream to affect distant sites this is a **hormonal** function. Although some authors classify the cytokines as short-range hormones, this chapter discusses hormones only in the classical context of relatively long range blood-circulating chemicals. The glands that produce them constitute the **endocrine** system. Endocrine glands contrast with **exocrine** glands (e.g. salivary glands), which release chemicals into ducts that connect to hollow organs, where the chemicals have their effect.

Some hormones are proteins or polypeptides (e.g. oxytocin, TSH, insulin). Others, while neither proteins nor polypeptides, are derivatives of amino acids (e.g. thyroxine, epinephrine). Others (steroids) are cholesterol derivatives.

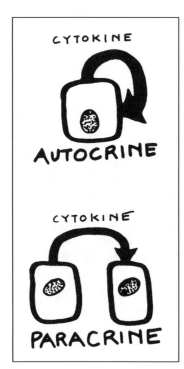

Figure 11-1

Hormones can act by affecting the activity of an enzyme, or the rate of synthesis of enzymes or other proteins. They may also act by affecting the permeability of cell membranes to molecules that affect cell function.

In general, the protein and polypeptide hormones, including epinephrine, interact with receptors on the cell surface. Specific cell receptors are important to ensure that the hormone acts only on specifically designated cells. Once having reacted with a specific cell surface receptor, this stimulates a second messenger within the cell to regulate cell activity. For most protein and polypeptide hormones the second messenger is cyclic AMP. Other messengers include cyclic GMP, inositol triphosphate, diglyceride, and calcium.

The steroid hormones act on cytoplasmic receptors, and the resulting complex moves to the nucleus to influence DNA transcription of proteins. Thyroid hormone directly enters the nucleus where it alters DNA, causing production of certain enzymes. A particular chemical may have more than one receptor type. Epinephrine, for instance, acts on alpha receptors, to produce vasoconstriction, and on beta receptors, to produce vasodilation.

Fig. 11-2. The endocrine glands.

Apart from the hormones produced in the pituitary, pineal, thyroid, parathyroid, pancreas, adrenals, pancreas, ovary and testis, there are other hormones that do not have their own personal glands, but are nonetheless hormones. Gastrin, secretin, and cholecystokinin, for instance, which are discussed in the GI chapter, are blood circulating hormones that are secreted by the digestive tract wall (Fig. 10-2). Erythropoetin is produced in the kidney. Prostaglandins are a diverse group of chemicals that are released from many tissues of the body and have many local and systemic functions, sometimes opposite to one another, e.g. causing vasoconstriction or vasodilation.

SPECIFIC HORMONES

GROWTH HORMONE (GH, **somatotropin**):
    ORIGIN: Anterior pituitary gland (acidophil cells)
    STRUCTURE: Polypeptide
    REGULATED BY: GH-releasing hormone (GHRH) and inhibiting hormone (somatostatin) from the hypothalamus.
    FUNCTION: Promotes growth of bone and cartilage; increases protein synthesis throughout the body; promotes lipid breakdown to fatty acids, which can be use for energy; decreases the use of glucose as an energy

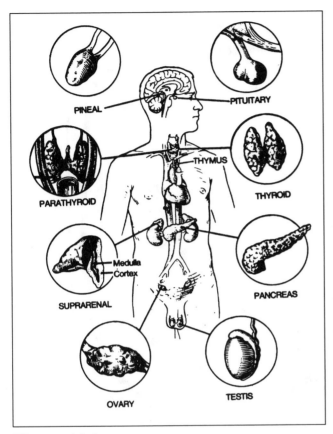

Figure 11-2

source, which raises blood glucose concentration and results in increased glycogen storage. GH appears to act indirectly by first inducing the liver to produce **somatomedins,** protein growth factors. Decreased blood levels of glucose or amino acids, as might occur in malnutrition, stimulate the pituitary to secrete GH, thereby restoring lost tissue proteins.

Another hormone, **somatomammotropin,** is produced by the placenta and resembles somatotropin in structure and function. By increasing maternal blood levels of glucose and fatty acids, somatomammotropin increases the availability of nutrients for the fetus.

EXCESS: Causes **gigantism** (symmetric) in children, and **acromegaly** (asymmetric growth and marked enlargement of hands, feet, forehead, jaw and other tissues) in adults.

DEFICIENCY: In children, causes **symmetrical dwarfism** with normal intelligence.

Fig. 11-3. Feedback loops of the pituitary gland.

PROLACTIN:
ORIGIN: Anterior pituitary gland (acidophil cells)
STRUCTURE: Protein

REGULATED BY: Prolactin-releasing and, especially, inhibiting hormone (PIF, prolactin inhibitory factor) from hypothalamus, which in turn are regulated by neural feedback to the hypothalamus during nursing.

FUNCTION: Stimulates milk secretion in pregnancy.
NOTE: **Estrogen** stimulates development of the breast duct system, breast fat deposition, and breast stroma; **progesterone** stimulates the development of breast glandular tissue and alveoli, the secretory structures of the breast; **prolactin** stimulates milk secretion into the alveoli during pregnancy and nursing, whereas **oxytocin** stimulates breast myoepithelial cells to contract, thereby externally ejecting the milk that has been stored in the breast alveoli.

EXCESS: May occur in prolactin-producing tumors, or with excess thyroid releasing hormone (TRH) production, which stimulates prolactin secretion in addition to TSH secretion. Galactorrhea (excess milk secretion) results, as well as amenorrhea and anovulation secondary to disturbances of the menstrual cycle. Nursing also stimulates prolactin production and hence is associated with decreased fertility during the phase of nursing. Excess prolactin in males results in testosterone deficiency and impotence.

ADRENOCORTICOTROPHIC HORMONE (ACTH, corticotropin)
ORIGIN: Anterior pituitary gland (basophil cells)
STRUCTURE: Polypeptide
REGULATED BY: Corticotropin releasing hormone (CRH) from hypothalamus, which in turn is regulated by negative feedback from blood levels of cortisol to both the hypothalamus (decreasing CRH secretion) and anterior pituitary gland (decreasing ACTH secretion). In addition, stress itself, whether physical or mental, can trigger CRH release through neural communication to the hypothalamus.

FUNCTION: Stimulates secretion of cortisol (a glucocorticoid) and also, to some degree, aldosterone (a mineralocorticoid) and androgenic steroids in the adrenal cortex.

EXCESS: **Cushing's disease** specifically refers to the clinical effects of increased ACTH secretion (and hence secondarily increased adrenal corticosteroid production) from a pituitary tumor. **Cushing's syndrome** is a broader term, referring to the results of excess corticosteroids, whether it be due to a primary oversecretion by the pituitary or adrenal, or chronic administration of corticosteroids (the most common cause). As a result of the increased output of **glucocorticoids,** there are obesity, buffalo hump deformity, moon-face, stria, osteoporosis, myopathy, psychosis, and diabetes from abnormalities in the metabolism and distribution of carbohydrates, proteins, and fats. The antiinflammatory effect of the glucocorticoids adds the symptoms of decreased inflammatory response. The ex-

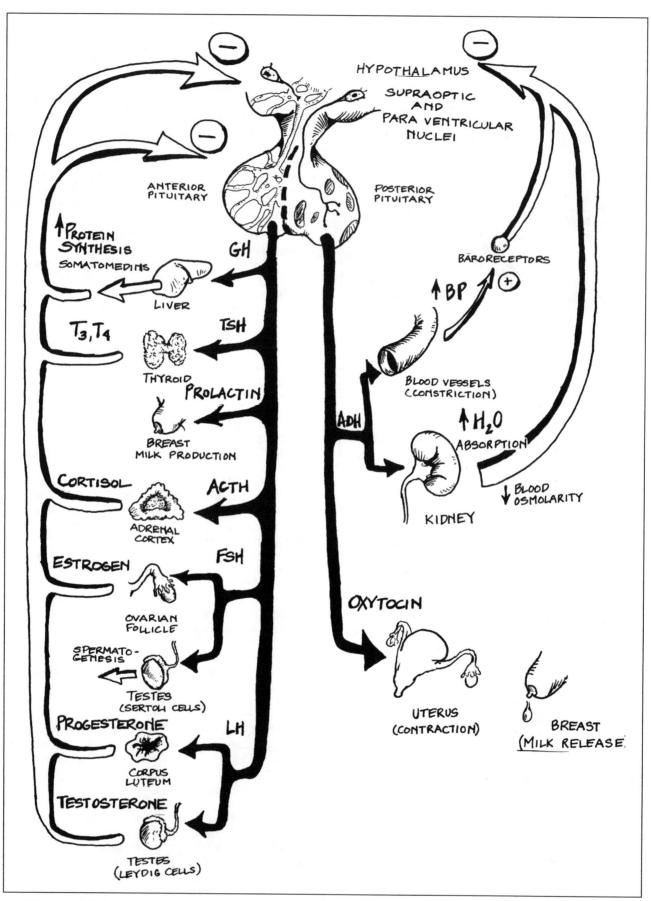

Figure 11-3

CHAPTER 11. THE ENDOCRINE SYSTEM

cess production of **mineralocorticoids** adds the symptoms of hypertension and hypokalemic alkalosis. The coinciding effects of increased **androgen** production include amenorrhea, hirsuitism, and acne. No wonder the patient has, on top of all this, stress ulcers—and polycythemia (excess red cell concentration), too.

DEFICIENCY: Although pituitary disease may be a cause of adrenal cortical deficiency (**Addison's disease**), most cases result from destruction of the adrenal cortex. Lack of aldosterone results in fluid loss that may cause hypotension, even shock and death, hyponatremia (decreased plasma sodium), hyperkalemia (high plasma potassium), and acidosis from inability of sodium to be reabsorbed in the kidney in exchange for $H+$. Loss of cortisol results in muscle weakness and poor tolerance to stress, from general inability to promote gluconeogenesis and protein and fat breakdown. Increased skin pigmentation occurs in Addison's disease of adrenal destruction, possibly due to the feedback increase in ACTH, which resembles melanocyte stimulating hormone in structure and has some effect in increasing skin pigmentation. The pigmentary effect is absent in Addison's disease of pituitary origin.

LUTEINIZING HORMONE (LH) AND FOLLICLE STIMULATING HORMONE (FSH)
ORIGIN: Anterior pituitary gland (basophil cells)
STRUCTURE: Glycoproteins
REGULATED BY: Hypothalamic gonadotrophic releasing hormone (GnRH), a releasing hormone for both LH and FSH. In males, GnRH is regulated by negative feedback from blood levels of testosterone. Also, spermatogenesis is believed to decrease FSH secretion in the pituitary through **inhibin**, a protein hormone produced by the Sertoli cells of the testes. In females, inhibin is produced by the corpus luteum and, together with estrogen and progesterone inhibit the production of LH and FSH through interactions with the pituitary gland and hypothalamus.
FUNCTION: In males, *L*H stimulates testosterone synthesis in the testes **Leydig** cells, whereas *FS*H stimulates *S*permatogenesis, facilitated by testes **Sertoli** cells. Mnemonic: FSH (fish) stimulates production of sperm (which swim like fish). (The Sertoli cells do not acutally produce sperm but facilitate the transformation of spermatids to spermatozoa. Futher maturation and motility of the spermatozoa occur on contact with the fluids of the epididymis, vas deferens, seminal vesicles, prostate gland, and bulbourethral glands. The alkalinity of the prostatic secretions, especially, contribute to activating sperm motility.)
In females, FSH, as the name implies, stimulates ovarian **follicles** to grow and produce estradiol. LH, as the name implies, stimulates the follicle to ovulate and mature into a **corpus luteum**, which secretes both estrogen and progesterone (Fig. 11-8).

THYROID STIMULATING HORMONE (TSH) (Fig. 11-3,11-4)
ORIGIN: Anterior pituitary (basophil cells)
STRUCTURE: Glycoprotein
REGULATION: Secretion is stimulated by hypothalamic TRH (thyrotropin-releasing hormone). In addition, thyroid hormone appears to act directly on the anterior pituitary TSH-secreting cells (and perhaps to some degree indirectly on hypothalamic TSH secretion) to suppress secretion.
FUNCTION: Controls production of thyroid hormone. Thyroid hormone is stored in the form of **thyroglobulin**, a glycoprotein, in the colloid of thyroid follicles (Fig. 11-4). TSH stimulates all aspects of thyroid hormone synthesis, including the uptake of iodide, its incorporation into thyroglobulin, and the breakdown of thyroglobulin to release thyroxine (T4) and triiodothyronine (T3), the active forms of thyroid hormone, which enter the blood stream. TSH also stimulates the proliferation of the thyroglobulin-synthesizing cuboidal cells of the thyroid follicles, thereby contributing to **goiter** (enlarged thyroid) in cases of excess TSH production. Once in the blood stream, T3 and T4 combine with, and are transported by a glycoprotein, **thyroxine-binding globulin (TBG)**. It is only the free-circulating hormone, as opposed to the TBG-bound portion that is metabolically active and directly enters cells. Thus, measurement of free T4 is a more reliable index of thyroid hormone function than measurement of total serum T4, which includes the TBG fraction.

Fig. 11-4. Synthesis of thyroid hormone.

MELANOCYTE STIMULATING HORMONE
ORIGIN: Anterior lobe of pituitary
STRUCTURE: Peptide
FUNCTION: Promotes melanin pigmentation of the skin

HYPOTHALAMIC RELEASING HORMONES:
ORIGIN: Hypothalamus
STRUCTURE: Peptides
FUNCTION: Stimulate release of hormones by the anterior pituitary.

ANTIDIURETIC HORMONE (ADH; vasopressin)
ORIGIN: Hypothalamus (stored in axon endings in posterior pituitary)
STRUCTURE: Polypeptide
REGULATED BY: Osmotic changes in blood (Na+); neural input to hypothalamus.
FUNCTION: Acts on the kidney to promote reabsorption of water into the blood circulation; a potent vasoconstrictor.
EXCESS: Fluid retention; hyponatremia.

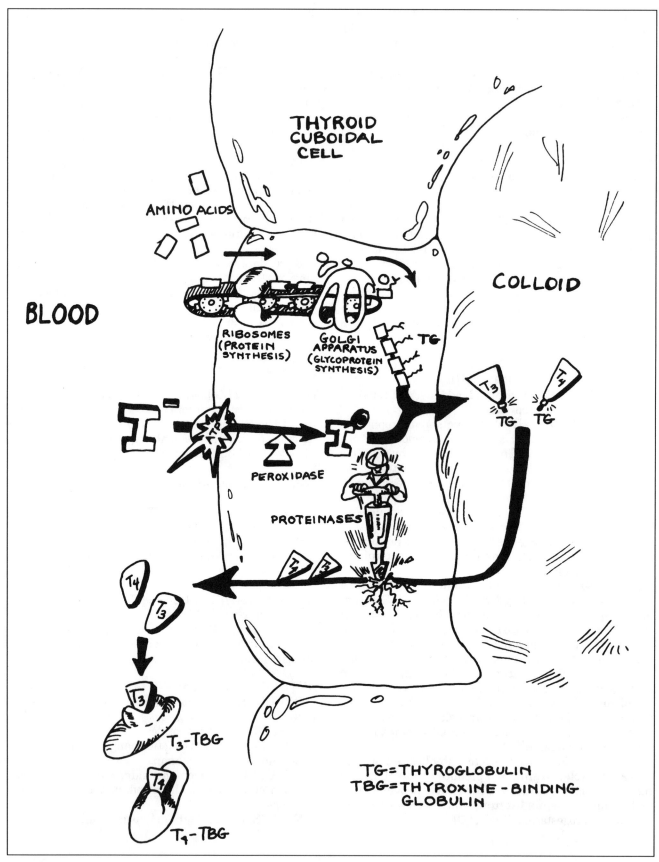

Figure 11-4

DEFICIENCY: Markedly increased thirst and urination. With severe ADH deficiency (**diabetes insipidus**), the patient may urinate 20 liters/day and drink 20 liters of water to compensate for the loss.

OXYTOCIN:

ORIGIN: Hypothalamus (stored in posterior pituitary)

STRUCTURE: Polypeptide

REGULATED BY: Sucking reflex communicated via hypothalamus.

FUNCTION: Stimulates uterine contraction; stimulates ejection of milk in lactating women.

MELATONIN:

ORIGIN: Pineal gland

STRUCTURE: Derivative or tryptophan and serotonin

FUNCTION: May have a role in regulating adrenal and gonadal functioning.

THYROID HORMONE—T4 (thyroxine) and T3 (triiodothyronine) (Fig. 11-4):

ORIGIN: Thyroid gland

STRUCTURE: Amino acid derivative of tyrosine

REGULATED BY: TSH

FUNCTION: Increases body metabolic rate by increasing protein, particularly enzyme, synthesis through increased DNA transcription to RNA.

EXCESS: **Hyperthyroidism (Grave's Disease)** includes increased metabolism, increased heart rate, nervousness, weight loss, goiter (thyroid gland enlargement), and exophthalmos (protruding eyes). Although elevated TSH levels can cause hyperthyroidism, in most cases TSH levels are low, indicating a primary cause in the thyroid gland from which excess thyroid hormone feeds back to the pituitary to decrease TSH levels. In most cases, the cause of hyperthyroidism appears to be an abnormal antibody (**LATS, long-acting thyroid stimulator**) that acts like TSH and stimulates the thyroid gland to produce thyroid hormone. Antibody to retroorbital tissues appears to be a factor in the development of exophthalmos.

Hyperthyroidism can be diagnosed by measuring blood levels of free thyroxine, the active form that is unattached to thyroid-binding globulin. One may also measure an increased uptake of radioactive iodide by the thyroid gland. Treatment may consist of removal of part of the thyroid, whether surgically or by administration of radioactive iodine-131 to ablate thyroid tissue. Alternatively one can use medications that block thyroid hormone synthesis (e.g. propylthiouracil, which blocks peroxidase activity).

DEFICIENCY: **Hypothyroidism** results in **cretinism** in children (dwarfism, enlarged tongue and abdomen and mental retardation). In adults, hypothyroidism results in weakness, decreased mentation, decreased tendon reflexes, cold intolerance and **myxedema** (non-pitting edema from, for some unclear reason, mucopolysaccharide deposition; thick, dry skin; puffy face). Thyroid hormone stimulates the breakdown of fats for energy utilization. Thus, hypothyroidism is also associated with fat accumulation and is a cause of hypercholesterolemia. Goiter may also occur with hypothyroidism, when TSH is elevated. (The increase in TSH results from lack of the normal suppression of TSH production by T3 and T4 feedback to the hypothalamus.)

Laboratory diagnostic tests of hypothyroidism include not only basal metabolic rate, radioactive iodide uptake and measurement of blood thyroid hormone levels, but measurement of TSH levels. Low TSH levels suggest a primary problem of decreased functioning at the hypothalamic-pituitary level. High TSH levels suggests a primary thyroid deficiency, with lack of suppressor feedback to the pituitary gland.

Thyroid hormone replacement is important in the treatment of hypothyroidism, but it is important to note that nutritional deficiency of dietary iodide is one of the causes of hypothyroidism. This cause is fortunately less common today, because iodide is added as a supplement to table salt.

PARATHYROID HORMONE (PTH)

ORIGIN: Parathyroid glands (four glands that lie posterior to the thyroid gland)

STRUCTURE: Polypeptide

REGULATION: Decreased blood calcium stimulates PTH secretion.

FUNCTION: Increases blood **calcium** levels by stimulating bone breakdown, and kidney and intestinal absorption of calcium. Although PTH also increases entry of **phosphate** into the blood from bone absorption, blood phosphate levels decrease, because PTH stimulates renal **excretion** of phosphate. This contrasts with vitamin D, which promotes increases in both calcium and phosphate levels in the blood, through bone absorption, renal reabsorption and intestinal absorption.

EXCESS: Hypercalcemia, and usually hypophosphatemia, with bone fractures and cysts, and tissue deposition of calcium.

DEFICIENCY: Hypocalcemia with **tetany**: Spastic contractions, particularly of wrist and ankle joints (**carpopedal spasm**) with convulsions and laryngeal spasm.

VITAMIN D

ORIGIN: Cholecalciferol (vitamin D3) is formed in the **skin** in response to ultraviolet light. Vitamin D3 is converted in the **liver** to 25-hydroxycholecalciferol, which is converted in the **kidney** to the active form of vitamin D, 1,25-hydroxycholecalciferol. Although termed a vitamin, it is actually a hormone, as it is synthesized in the skin (from cholesterol), apart from being ingested in the diet.

STRUCTURE: Steroid

REGULATION: Vitamin D levels increase through dietary intake of vitamin D and through exposure to ultraviolet light. Also, parathyroid hormone is necessary for the conversion in the kidney of 25-hydroxycholecalciferol to 1,25-hydroxycholecalciferol.

FUNCTION: Promotes the absorption of calcium from the intestines and kidneys. In large amounts, vitamin D promotes absorption of calcium from bone to blood, but in smaller amounts, vitamin D promotes bone calcification, the context in which one usually thinks of vitamin D.

EXCESS: Hypercalcemia and renal stones.

DEFICIENCY: Causes hypocalcemia and hypophosphatemia, with resultant **rickets** (bending with poor calcification of developing bone in children) or **osteomalacia** (decalcification and softening of bones in adults). In both of these there is impaired mineralization. These should be distinguished from another condition, **osteoporosis**, in which there is reduction in bone mass as a whole, rather than select reduction of the mineral content.

CALCITONIN (thyrocalcitonin):

ORIGIN: Thyroid ("C" cells)

STRUCTURE: Peptide

REGULATION: Increased blood calcium increases calcitonin secretion.

FUNCTION: Its net effect is opposite to that of parathyroid hormone, but it is not nearly as potent. It mildly decreases plasma calcium. Calcitonin acts on bone by decreasing the activity of osteoclasts (cells that break down bone).

EPINEPHRINE AND NOREPINEPHRINE:

ORIGIN: Adrenal medulla

STRUCTURE: Derivative of tyrosine.

REGULATED BY: Neural input to adrenal medulla.

FUNCTION: Epinephrine, and to some degree norepinephrine, stimulate glycogen breakdown, lipid breakdown, and gluconeogenesis (the opposite of insulin). **NoR**epinephrine, present in sympathetic nerve endings, has ge**NeR**al vasoconstrictive effects, by interacting with blood vessel alpha-1 receptors. Epinephrine vasoconstricts too, but not in all places. Like norepinephrine, epinephrine vasoconstricts at blood vessel alpha-1 receptors, but vasodilates at blood vessel beta-2 receptors, most notably those in skeletal muscle and heart, thereby facilitating blood perfusion during a flight-or-fight response. The adrenal medulla produces more epinephrine than norepinephrine. Norepinephrine, though, is the neurotransmitter in postganglionic axons of the sympathetic nervous system, where it par-

ticularly mediates catabolic (energy-expending; "flight-or-fight") responses.

EXCESS: Hypertension and tachycardia.

Fig. 11-5. Hormonal relations of the adrenal gland.

GLUCOCORTICOIDS (especially cortisol):

ORIGIN: Adrenal cortex

STRUCTURE: Steroid

REGULATION: Secretion stimulated by ACTH. Physical or mental stress can increase ACTH secretion and hence cortisol secretion.

FUNCTION: Mobilize carbohydrates, lipids, and proteins during periods of stress, by elevating blood glucose, fatty acids, and amino acids (Fig. 11-7). It does so in part by stimulating gluconeogenesis in the liver. Also, it promotes breakdown of fats in adipose tissue to energy-providing fatty acids. Glucocorticoids also promote the breakdown of proteins, in tissues other than the liver. The resulting increase in blood amino acids provide a source for synthesizing glucose and other molecules in the liver.

Glucocorticoids also are antiinflammatory: they inhibit histamine secretion, inhibit lymphocyte production, and stabilize macrophage lysosomes. In a sense, the antiinflammatory action is a therapeutic response to the "stress" of the inflammatory process, which in itself can be harmful to the body. Glucocorticoids also increase gastric acid production.

EXCESS: Cushing's syndrome (see effects of excess ACTH). Many of the effects have to do with glucorticoid influence on the metabolism and body distribution of fats, carbohydrates and proteins.

DEFICIENCY: Addison's Disease (hyponatremia, hypotension, increased skin pigmentation, muscle weakness) most commonly arising from autoimmune destruction of the adrenal cortices (see signs of ACTH deficiency).

MINERALOCORTICOIDS (aldosterone being most important):

ORIGIN: Adrenal cortex

REGULATION: Secretion is stimulated by ACTH and by the renin/angiotensin axis. Renin stimulates conversion of the protein angiotensinogen to angiotensin I, which then becomes angiotensin II. Angiotensin II stimulates the synthesis and release of aldosterone by the adrenal cortex. In addition, elevated blood potassium stimulates adrenal aldosterone secretion whereas elevated sodium decreases secretion.

STRUCTURE: Steroid

FUNCTION: Stimulates kidney reabsorption of sodium into the circulation, with exchange for potassium.

EXCESS: May be primary, the effect of primary adrenal hyperplasia (**Conn's syndrome**; **primary hyperaldosteronism**); or secondary to excess renin

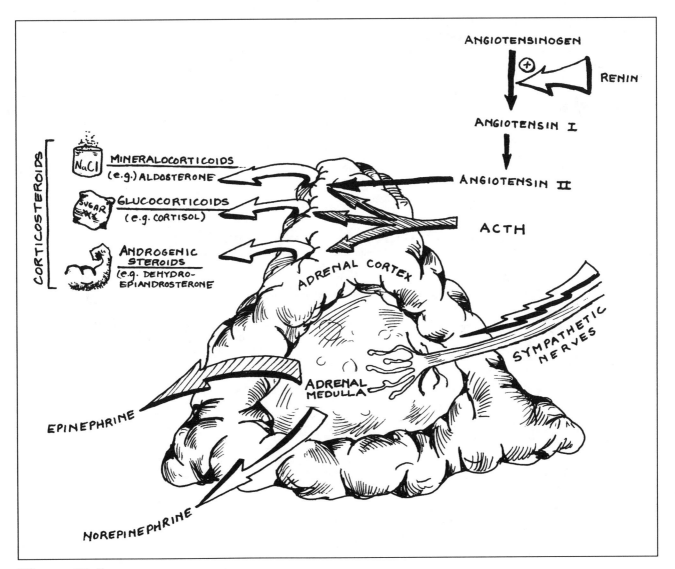

Figure 11-5

(**secondary hyperaldosteronism**), which may occur with renin-producing juxtaglomerular cell tumors or other kind of renal disorders. There are fluid retention, hypertension, and potassium loss (hypokalemia) with associated muscle weakness. Aldosterone, in addition to promoting potassium exchange for sodium, also promotes exchange of H+ for sodium. Hence, hyperaldosteronism may also be associated with an alkalosis.

DEFICIENCY: May result from adrenal destruction. Moreover, since aldosterone secretion is stimulated both by ACTH and by angiotensin II, deficiency may result from either a decrease in ACTH or a deficiency of the renin-angiotensin system. There are fluid and sodium loss (perhaps even shock from decreased blood volume), and potassium elevation (hyperkalemia) with associated cardiac arrhythmias.

INSULIN:
   ORIGIN: Beta cells of pancreas
   STRUCTURE: Polypeptide
   REGULATION: Secretion is stimulated by increased blood glucose concentration. An excess of certain amino acids also stimulates insulin secretion, which in turn clears the blood of excess amino acids by promoting the entry of certain amino acids into cells.
   FUNCTION: Facilitates the uptake of blood glucose by cells for storage as glycogen (particularly in the liver and muscle); synthesis of protein (insulin also increases

amino acid uptake by cells); synthesis of fatty acids in the liver, which are transported via VLDL lipoproteins to adipose cells, where they are stored as triglycerides. Or, the glucose may be utilized for energy or other cell functions. Insulin inhibits gluconeogenesis (formation of glucose). Insulin does not influence glucose uptake in the brain. Rather, glucose can enter brain cells without insulin. This is a good thing, as the brain requires glucose for fuel and would otherwise be terribly deprived if insulin levels were lacking; unlike other tissues, the brain cannot use fatty acids for fuel, as fatty acids do not cross the blood-brain barrier. That is why hypoglycemia is frequently accompanied by nervousness and even loss of consciousness.

EXCESS: **Hypoglycemia** (decreased blood glucose; nervousness, dizziness).

DEFICIENCY: **Diabetes mellitus**: elevated blood glucose, polyuria (increased urination), polydipsia (increased water intake), fatigue, coma, hyperlipidemia.

Fig. 11-6. The effects of insulin on energy utilization. The presence or absence of insulin helps to decide

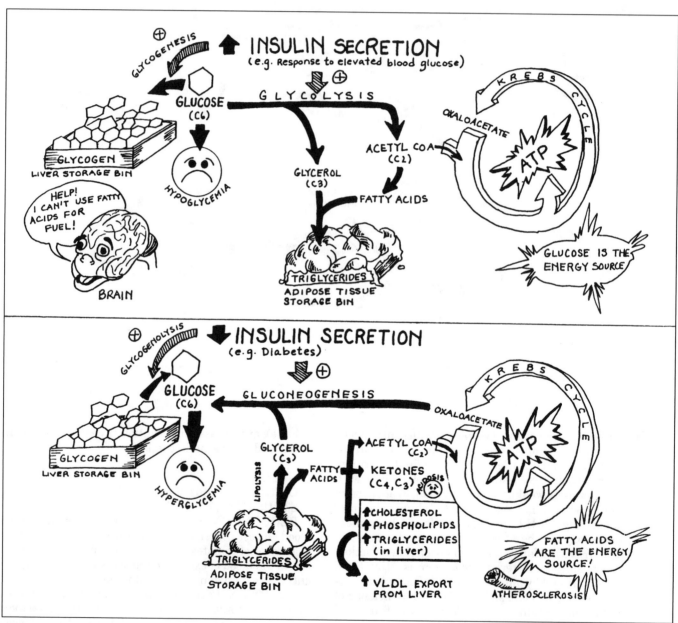

Figure 11-6

whether carbohydrates or lipids will be the main source of energy. When blood glucose is high, this stimulates the pancreas to secrete insulin. Insulin then drives the excess glucose into cells, where it can be stored as glycogen (glycogenesis) or broken down (glycolysis) and used in the Krebs cycle to generate ATP as an energy source. Meanwhile, fatty acids are stored as triglycerides in adipose tissue.

When blood glucose is low, insulin levels decrease. Then, adipose tissue trigyceride stores break down to form fatty acids, which are utilized as the energy source in the Krebs cycle, while glycogen breakdown and gluconeogenesis are stimulated, thereby restoring the low glucose levels. Maintaining adequate glucose levels is vital, since the brain relies on glucose as its sole source of energy.

A lack of insulin (or insulin receptors) occurs in diabetes mellitus. Concurrent with the breakdown of adipose tissue triglycerides to fatty acids, some of the excess fatty acids which do not enter the Krebs cycle are diverted to form ketones, such as acetoacetic acid, causing an acidosis, whereas some form excess cholesterol, phospholipids, and triglycerides in the liver, which incorporates these lipids into VLDL lipoproteins for export into the blood stream. The elevated lipids are associated with an increased risk of eventually developing atherosclerosis.

Fig. 11-7. Hormonal effects on carbohydrate, lipid and protein metabolism.

GLUCAGON:
 ORIGIN: Alpha cells of pancreas
 STRUCTURE: Polypeptide
 REGULATION: Secretion inhibited by increased blood glucose concentration. An excess of certain amino acids stimulates glucagon secretion (in keeping with glucagon's effect in promoting amino acid uptake by liver cells).
 FUNCTION: Stimulates glycogen breakdown and gluconeogenesis in the liver, thereby increasing blood glucose levels. These effects are opposite to those of insulin, but glucagon resembles insulin in that both promote uptake of amino acids by liver cells.
 EXCESS: Found in glucagon-secreting tumors (**glucaconomas**). The patient may develop diabetes mellitus, as well as a strange skin rash called **necrolytic migratory erythema**.

SOMATOSTATIN:
 ORIGIN: Delta cells of pancreas; hypothalamus
 STRUCTURE: Peptide

 REGULATION: Glucose, fatty acids, amino acids, cholecystokinin, vasoactive intestinal peptide and glucagon stimulate somatostatin secretion.
 FUNCTION: In the hypothalamus, somatostatin inhibits growth hormone secretion. Pancreatic somatostatin inhibits digestion and use of absorbed nutrients in a number of ways. It inhibits gastrointestinal motility, inhibits secretion of HCL and a number of digestive enzymes in the stomach, small intestine and pancreas, and inhibits absorption of glucose and triglycerides in the intestine. In the pancreas, it also inhibits insulin and glucagon secretion (a very negative-dispositioned chemical). It may function as a negative feedback from excess intake of nutrients.
 EXCESS: Occurs with rare somatostatin-secreting tumors (somatostatinomas). The patient develops diabetes mellitus, malabsorption and weight loss.

ESTROGENS (estradiol being the most important) (Fig. 11-8)
 ORIGIN: Ovary
 STRUCTURE: Steroid
 REGULATED BY: FSH
 FUNCTION: Necessary for development of the breasts (ducts and fat), female sex organs and secondary female characteristics. Needed for proliferation of the uterine endometrium during the early (preovulatory, or proliferative) phase of the menstrual cycle. When used in birth control pills, estrogens function in part to prevent ovulation by preventing a rise in LH and FSH. Also, estrogens thicken the cervical mucus, making it less receptive to sperm, and inhibit implantation of the ovum in the endometrium.
 EXCESS: Used as a birth control measure. There is a small increased risk of thromboembolic and cerebrovascular disease and possibly carcinoma of the cervix; there may be menstrual bleeding abnormalities and an increased risk of headache, hypertension, and elevated blood glucose and triglycerides. Postmenopausal use may decrease the risk of arteriosclerosis through decreasing LDL cholesterol levels and raising HDL levels, in addition to relieving menopausal symptoms, including hot flushes, decreased vaginal lubrication, and osteoporosis. There may be an increased risk of endometrial cancer and continued growth of uterine fibroids, which normally regress after menopause.
 DEFICIENCY: Menopausal symptoms: amenorrhea, hot flushes, thin vaginal mucosa with decreased vaginal lubrication; osteoporosis.

PROGESTERONE (Fig. 11-8):
 ORIGIN: Corpus luteum of the ovary
 STRUCTURE: Steroid
 REGULATED BY: LH

HORMONE	EFFECT ON CARBOHYDRATES	EFFECT ON LIPIDS	EFFECT ON PROTEINS
INSULIN Majors Aims: Clear blood of excess glucose; use the excess glucose, not fatty acids, as energy source; store some of excess glucose as glycogen.	Clears the blood of glucose by promoting entry of glucose into cells, especially liver, muscle and adipose cells (but not brain). Inhibits gluconeogenesis. Promotes use of glucose as energy source. Promotes storage of excess glucose as glycogen, and as triglycerides through fatty acid synthesis in liver and export to adipose tissue as triglycerides via VLDL.	Promotes fatty acid synthesis in the liver and storage as triglycerides in adipose tissue.	Promotes entry of amino acids into cells, and protein synthesis. Inhibits protein breakdown.
GLUCAGON Majors Aims: Protect against too low a blood glucose, by raising blood glucose.	Increases blood glucose concentration by increasing glycogen breakdown and increasing gluconeogenesis.	Increases trigyceride breakdown to fatty acids	Increases amino acid uptake in liver for gluconeogenesis
GROWTH HORMONE Major aims: promote protein synthesis; use fatty acids, not glucose, as fuel.	Decreases use of glucose by cells (except for brain), resulting in increased blood glucose (unlike insulin) concentration and increased glycogen synthesis in the liver (similar to insulin).	Promotes lipid breakdown in adipose tissue to fatty acids as energy source.	Increases uptake of many amino acids by cells throughout body. Promotes protein synthesis. Prevents protein breakdown.
EPINEPHRINE Majors aims: Break down glycogen and fat to supply glucose and fatty acids	Increases glycogen breakdown to glucose	Breaks down triglycerides to fatty acids.	
CORTISOL Major aims: mobilize carbohydrates, lipids, and proteins for use during stress.	Increases blood glucose concentration. Decreases use of glucose by cells; stimulates gluconeogenesis in liver	Increases blood fatty acid concentration. Promotes lipid breakdown in adipose tissue to fatty acids as energy source.	Increases blood amino acid concentration. Decreases amino acid entry into extrahepatic cells and moves amino acids out of extrahepatic cells to be available in liver for gluconeogenesis. Increases liver protein synthesis but elsewhere decreases protein synthesis and increases protein breakdown. Increases conversion of amino acids to glucose, in liver cells.

Figure 11-7

FUNCTION: Prepares the endometrium to receive the fertilized egg during the postovulatory (progestational) phase of the menstrual cycle.

EXCESS: Long-acting injectable progestins may be used for contraception. They interfere with ovulation and may cause menstrual bleeding irregularities.

TESTOSTERONE:
  ORIGIN: Testes
  STRUCTURE: Steroid
  REGULATED BY: LH
  FUNCTION: Development of male genitalia, male secondary sex characteristics, spermatogenesis, and libido. Androgens also promote skeletal and muscular development.

EXCESS: In children, a testicular testosterone-secreting tumor may cause premature sexual development. The child may also be relatively short, because testosterone, while promoting bone growth, also promotes closure of the bone epiphysial growth plates, thereby shortening the time of increased growth. The administration of synthetic androgens in adult athletes will promote muscular development, but at the risk of developing concurrent abnormal liver function and decreased testicular production of sperm and testosterone. In women, there may be abnormalities of the menstrual cycle, in addition to hirsuitism and other masculinizing effects.

DEFICIENCY: Results in impotence. When deficiency begins in early childhood, there may be failure of development of male secondary sex characteristics.

CHORIONIC GONADOTROPHIN (HCG):
  ORIGIN: Chorion and placenta
  STRUCTURE: Glycoprotein
  FUNCTION: Prevents the corpus luteum from involuting in pregnancy, allowing a rise of estrogen and progesterone. Stimulates testosterone production in the testes of the male fetus.

The Menstrual Cycle and Pregnancy

Prior to puberty, which usually occurs between ages 11 and 15 in girls, there are no menstrual cycles, as the production of FSH and LH is insufficient. Both FSH and LH are necessary for the proper preparation of the uterus for pregnancy. FSH stimulates the growth of the ovarian follicles, which produce estrogen and release the ovum. LH triggers follicular ovulation and transformation of the follicle to a corpus luteum, which secretes both estrogen and progesterone.

Fig. 11-8. The menstrual cycle. The sequence of events in the menstrual cycle are as follows:

1) The normal menstrual cycle, on the average, occurs about once every 28 days. Day 1 of the menstrual cycle coincides with the onset of **menstruation**, which usually lasts about 4-5 days. **FSH** during this time stimulates the ovarian follicles to mature and produce estrogen, which then induces **proliferation** of the uterine endometrium. (Actually a group of follicles enlarge at the beginning of the cycle, but after the fifth or sixth day, a single one of them grows to reach a size of about 2 cm, whereas the others degenerate.) In addition to estrogen secretion, the mature follicle contains the ovum to be fertilized after ovulation. Days 1-13 of the cycle are referred to as the **follicular, or proliferative phase** of the cycle.

2) In the usual 28-day menstrual cycle, ovulation occurs about day 14. A menstrual cycle, though, may normally be 21-35 days long. Usually, regardless of the length of the menstrual cycle, ovulation occurs about 14 days **prior** to menstruation. Just prior to ovulation there is an increase in estrogen and, to some degree, progesterone, coinciding with the follicular maturation.

The estrogen, in addition to its effects on uterine proliferation, triggers a sudden increase in the pituitary production of LH and FSH, particularly LH. (The direct stimulus to both LH and FSH secretion is hypothalamic gonadotropin releasing hormone, GnRH. A peculiarity of this arrangement is that GnRH must be released from the hypothalamus in **pulses**. Continuous administration of GnRH will not stimulate FSH and LH secretion.) The surge in LH secretion induces **ovulation**, i.e. the release of the ovum, which then begins it's trip into the peritoneal cavity, Fallopian tubes, and uterus.

3) The increase in LH production stimulates not only ovulation but the development of the corpus luteum, which produces not only estrogen, but significant amounts of progesterone. Progesterone causes the uterus to enter a new phase beyond the proliferative stage, the **luteal phase**, in which there are endometrial **secretory gland development** and secretion, to prepare the uterine endometrium for implantation of the ovum, should the ovum be fertilized.

4) If fertilization does not occur, the increased estrogen and progesterone from the corpus luteum, and probably another luteal hormone, **inhibin**, feed back to the pituitary gland and hypothalamus, causing decreased LH and FSH production; the corpus luteum therefore can no longer be maintained and degenerates.

Estrogen itself appears to have a paradoxical effect on LH and FSH secretion, in that rising levels of estrogen in the early part of the cycle stimulate FSH and LH secretion, whereas chronic presence of estrogen supresses FSH secretion. The estrogen and progesterone in **birth control pills** act to suppress ovulation, mainly by inhibiting FSH and LH secretion. The dominant ovarian follicle can't develop without FSH and there is then no rising estogen to trigger the LH surge and ovulation. Excess progesterone also thickens the cervical mucus,

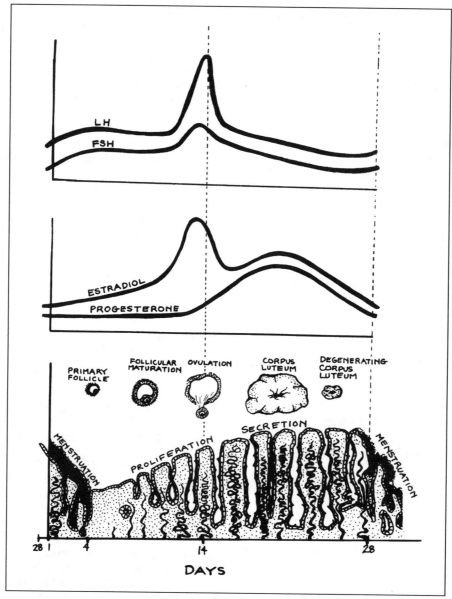

Figure 11-8

making it less receptive to sperm. It also decreases Fallopian tube motility.

Chronic excess progesterone also renders the endometrium atrophic, a reason why it is given in large amounts in **endometriosis**, to control the ectopic pathologic areas of endometrial development. In the **"morning-after"** pill, a large dose of estrogen and progesterone thickens the endometrium, which then sloughs on withdrawal of the hormones.

With degeneration of the corpus luteum in the normal menstrual cycle, estrogen and progesterone production decrease; the uterine endometrium can no longer be maintained, and sloughs (**menstruation**). (Menstrual blood normally does not clot, as the sloughing endometrium releases a fibrinolysin that inhibits clotting.) The decrease in estrogen and progesterone at this time is noted by the hypothalamus (as a decrease in negative estrogen and progesterone feedback), causing a renewal of LH and FSH production, thereby initiating a new menstrual cycle, which begins with growth of new ovarian follicles.

5) If fertilization occurs, it generally happens in the Fallopian tube. The ovum can be fertilized within only about a day after ovulation. Since sperm remain viable

for only about 1-3 days, intercourse must take place within about a day or so before or after ovulation for fertilization to occur. The trick is to know precisely when ovulation occurs, which is not always a simple matter. One index, although not absolutely reliable, is the rise in **basal body temperature**, which occurs just after ovulation and persists for the last half of the menstrual cycle. The fertilized egg reaches the uterus about 3-4 days after its fertilization in the lateral end of the Fallopian tube but does not implant in the endometrium until 3-5 days later.

6) Implantation causes the uterus to quickly produce **HCG (human chorionic gonadotrophin)**, a hormone that has effects similar to LH. This maintains the corpus luteum, ensuring a continuing supply of estrogen and progesterone during pregnancy and preventing the uterine endothelium from sloughing. Actually, the placenta itself is capable of estrogen and progesterone secretion in the latter 2 trimesters of pregnancy, so the corpus luteum is not needed in those times. The **placenta** develops from a fusion of embryonic and maternal tissue, along with a closely interdigitating blood supply that connects the maternal and fetal circulations via diffusion to and from the mother and fetus.

The rapid rise in HCG provides the basis for pregnancy testing. One can detect elevated HCG levels of pregnancy as early as 8 days after ovulation, even before the first missed period. HCG elevation peaks about 2 months into pregnancy, thereafter declining to reach a steady state that lasts from about 6 months to the end of pregnancy.

The primordial follicles gradually decrease in number through the years, eventually leading to **menopause**, where their disappearance means a decrease in the production of estrogen and progesterone.

GASTRIN (Fig. 10-2):
  ORIGIN: Gastric mucosa
  STRUCTURE: Polypeptide
  REGULATION: Secretion stimulated by vagus nerve, distension of duodenum, peptides. Secretion inhibited by secretin, Gastric Inhibitory Peptide, and excess acidity.
  FUNCTION: Activates secretion of gastric acid, pepsin, and intrinsic factor.
  EXCESS: Duodenal ulcers
SECRETIN (Fig. 10-2):
  ORIGIN: Duodenal and jejunal mucosa
  STRUCTURE: Peptide
  REGULATION: Stimulated by vagus nerve, direct contact with food, fat, and acid.
  FUNCTION: Inhibits gastric acid secretion; stimulates the pancreas to secrete water and bicarbonate; stimulates stomach pepsin secretion.

CHOLECYSTOKININ (pancreozymin)
  ORIGIN: Duodenal and jejunal mucosal cells
  STRUCTURE: Peptide
  REGULATION: Secretion stimulated by vagus nerve, direct contact with food, fat and acid.
  FUNCTION: Stimulates pancreatic secretion of enzymes and bicarbonate; stimulates gallbladder contraction. Decreases gastric motility.

INDEX